FOOT CARE
handbook

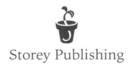

Storey Publishing

The mission of Storey Publishing is to serve our customers by
publishing practical information that encourages
personal independence in harmony with the environment.

Edited by Deborah Burns and Lisa H. Hiley
Art direction and book design by Ash Austin
Text production by Jennifer Jepson Smith
Indexed by Andrea Chesman
Back cover photo (author) by
© 2021 Stephanie Tourles
Illustrations by © Choo Chung

Text © 2021 by Stephanie L. Tourles
Portions of this book appeared in *Natural Foot
Care* (Storey Publishing, 1998).

This publication is intended to provide educational information for the reader on the covered subject. It is not intended to take the place of personalized medical counseling, diagnosis, and treatment from a trained health professional. Please consult a physician or other health professional if needed.

Storey books are available at special discounts when purchased in bulk for premiums and sales promotions as well as for fund-raising or educational use. Special editions or book excerpts can also be created to specification. For details, please call 800-827-8673, or send an email to sales@storey.com.

Storey Publishing
210 MASS MoCA Way
North Adams, MA 01247
storey.com

Printed in the United States by McNaughton &
Gunn
10 9 8 7 6 5 4 3 2 1

PRINTED IN USA
on Canadian paper

MIX
Paper
FSC FSC® C011935

Library of Congress Cataloging-in-Publication
Data on file

Dedicated to Myra Achorn, foot reflexology instructor extraordinaire.
I've had many teachers over the years, but you were the best!
You once told me, "Learning is a lifelong process, and reflexology will take you
on a journey that never really ends. It is a journey of healing and
self-discovery. When you follow your dreams, you open the door to
more possibilities than you can imagine. Learning can be fun,
but earning money doing something you love is even more fun!"

That has proved to be true!
I'm honored to have studied with you
and blessed to call you my friend.

CONTENTS

5 / Common Foot Problems, Uncommon Remedies   48

You Can Have Happy, Healthy Feet

I've been fascinated with feet since I was a youngster. Growing up in Stone Mountain, Georgia, I went barefoot whenever possible. My strong, tough feet enjoyed the sensory stimulation of the outdoor world. Much to the dismay of my mother, my soles were forever filthy: green from grass, black from tar, sticky from tree sap, or muddy from playing in the creek. Reminders to wash my feet before entering the house were constant, but I never listened.

My love for foot care began with watching my grandfather soak his aching, fatigued feet every night. He was a carpenter who also tended two big gardens and about two dozen cows, so his feet yearned for relief. He would fill an old dishpan with either warm or ice-cold water—depending on the season—to which he added, of all things, two tablespoons of Massengill douche powder! The blend of boric acid, alum powder, eucalyptus oil, thyme oil, menthol crystals, and methyl salicylate cooled, deodorized, and relaxed his feet, while easing pain. Foot soaks pulled the day's stresses right out of him, he told me.

My grandfather also lovingly cared for my grandmother's very narrow and always tender feet. She suffered from poor circulation and edema in her lower legs, and it didn't help that she always wore shoes that were too tight and too short and had two-inch heels. Grandfather would often give her feet and legs a comforting massage. I learned at a young age that foot care should be part of everyday life because neglected feet could negatively affect your entire body and outlook.

As I grew up, I learned from personal experience how injured, unhappy feet can make you miserable. Over the last two decades, I've suffered a broken toe, a sprained ankle, Morton's neuroma, plantar fasciitis, arthritis in my toe, and mild frostbite. I've dropped a bucket of water on one bare foot and had nine yellow-jacket stings on the other. Plus, I've had two major falls that severely altered my gait and created much foot pain (and ultimately two hip replacements!), so I know what people are suffering when their feet are in distress.

I love feet, and as a certified foot reflexologist, licensed massage therapist, and licensed aesthetician, I work with them nearly every day. When it comes to bodywork, I think feet are the best part of the body to work on. My clients would likely agree, as evidenced by their deep sighs of relief as I release the aches and tension from their hardworking, tired dogs. I target their feet with a comprehensive combination of reflexology, massage, Epsom salts foot soaks, herbal treatments, and aromatherapy, and I know I'm making their entire body feel better from the ground up.

I wrote this book to deliver much-needed education about keeping feet healthy and natural solutions to common foot woes. My hope is that reading these pages will give you a new respect for your feet and an understanding of their structure, function, and importance to overall comfort. If you ignore or mistreat your feet, life can be miserable, but if you make the conscious choice to care for them properly, your feet will thank you—as will your entire body!

Happy Feet = Happy You!

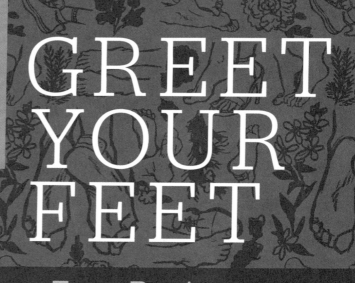

1 GREET YOUR FEET

Foot Basics

f our feet could speak, what might they say?

- Fashionista: "We're too confined in these tight, pointy shoes! Our arches are cramping, our heels are numb, and our toes are painful and deformed."
- Stylish businessperson: "Your slick Italian leather shoes and nylon dress socks are choking us. We look fabulous, but we can't breathe!"
- Active teenager: "These shoes smell so bad it's embarrassing."
- Busy parent with no time for self-care: "We have corns, calluses, and cracked heels. We ache. Give us a break!"

If our feet could speak, they'd probably complain, and loudly. Our feet walk, run, jump, skip, climb, balance, and grip, taking us where we need to go. It's tough to get along without them. But what do we do instead of keeping them in tip-top shape? We abuse them!

You're going to hear me say this more than once: Ill-fitting, poorly designed shoes are the primary source of most foot problems. We encase our feet in suffocating socks, pantyhose, or tights and stuff them into confining shoes. We buy shoes that are too small or have hard or inflexible soles that stress our feet. We choose exercise shoes with overly cushioned support, rigid stability, and elevated heels with turned-up toe boxes that don't allow our poor feet to move and spring as they are meant to do, so they weaken and deform over time. I feel so strongly about this issue that I nearly called this book *The Evils of Modern Footwear*!

Even when properly shod, feet may experience more wear and tear than any other body part and thus are more

FOOT NOTE

"My feet are killing me!" Sound familiar? Foot pain is one of the top reasons that folks over age 40 visit their healthcare provider. And the majority of sufferers are women, who have about four times as many foot problems as men. No surprise there, as "fashionable" women's shoes usually squeeze toes into submission or bend feet into unnatural shapes, causing any number of problems over time.

prone to discomfort and injury. They often also suffer from lack of effective hygiene and proper maintenance. How many people regularly scrub their feet, including the soles and between the toes, much less actually dry between the toes? Neglect and mistreatment can lead to myriad foot problems. Avoiding these issues just takes a little education. Let's start with some basics on the structure and function of your precious feet.

Your Amazing Foot

Leonardo da Vinci is reputed to have said, "The human foot is a masterpiece of engineering and a work of art." A normal foot contains 26 bones (or 28 if you count the two little sesamoid bones near the big toe joint) and 33 joints, plus more than 100 muscles, tendons, and ligaments and a complicated network of blood vessels and nerves.

The bones support the soft tissues and provide the flexible structure for functional movement, while the heel pad, the ball of the foot, and the arches act as shock absorbers, cushioning the jolts that occur with every step. Just walking around the office, going grocery shopping, or taking the dog around the block exerts several hundred tons of pressure on the feet.

In order for the feet to propel the body forward and absorb shock, the brain and spinal cord must first receive messages from the nerve endings located in the feet. The feet have thousands of sensory neurons (it's one of the highest concentrations of sensory neurons anywhere in the body), which makes them extremely sensitive to stimuli. These "earthward antennae," as I call them, send important information about the terrain and the body's positioning to the brain so that the brain can direct the feet to respond appropriately.

No two pairs of feet are identical, and even on the same person, feet usually differ slightly from each other. Foot shape and size, arch height, and length of toes all vary. Inherited traits may produce some characteristics, such as extremely high arches or particularly sweaty or odoriferous feet, that are potentially problematic.

FOOT NOTE
Your feet contain 25 percent of the bones in your entire body!

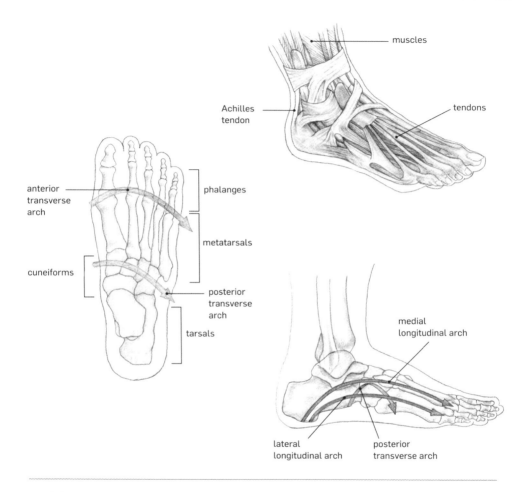

anterior transverse arch

phalanges

cuneiforms

metatarsals

posterior transverse arch

tarsals

muscles

tendons

Achilles tendon

medial longitudinal arch

lateral longitudinal arch

posterior transverse arch

FOOT NOTE

The Achilles tendon is the largest and strongest tendon in the entire body. It connects the two calf muscles to the heel bone. When the calf muscles flex, the Achilles tendon pulls on the heel, allowing us to rise onto our toes, as we do when running, jumping, walking, or reaching for something overhead.

Children's Unique Feet

Infant feet are not simply tiny versions of adult feet. They are primarily cartilage and not fully formed. As the feet grow and strengthen, the cartilage becomes bone, a process that continues into the late teens.

Baby feet tend to be a bit chubby, wider at the toes and tapering toward the heel. They normally appear flat because the arches aren't formed and the soles are protected with pads of fat. When a child first starts walking, these fat pads cause a waddling gait. (That's why we call them toddlers!) Children usually start taking adultlike, heel-to-toe steps around 3 to 4 years of age. The arches begin to develop when the child is about 2½ years old and don't fully form until 6 to 8 years of age.

Proper care for your child's feet is essential. The most important thing you can do is allow them to develop naturally and without constriction. Babies should be encouraged to stretch and kick their feet as much as possible to develop muscles and prepare their feet for standing and walking. They do not need shoes, just soft socks that don't bind. As your child grows, encourage them to go barefoot as often as possible, indoors and outdoors. This strengthens their feet, knees, legs, hips, and back.

Shoes need to fit properly, be extremely comfortable, allow plenty of wiggle room for toes, be super flexible, and have soft soles. Rigid shoes minimize the natural movement of feet and can result in problems down the road.

This category can include many fashionable dress shoes, boots, clogs, and sandals, as well as ultrapadded athletic shoes and most sports-specialized shoes. Please limit the time that your child spends wearing these styles, instead searching out brands that promote foot health. See Resources (page 126) for a few suggestions.

Toenails Are Part of Your Feet

Toenails are composed of keratin, the same protein that makes up your skin and hair, but in a harder and tougher version. They protect the ends of your toes and the bones and nerves lying underneath. Toenails grow approximately $\frac{1}{16}$ to $\frac{1}{8}$ inch (1.6 to 3 mm) per month, two to three times slower than fingernails. To grow an entirely new toenail takes 12 to 18 months. Toenails and fingernails grow fastest during hot weather, pregnancy, and teenage years.

Toenails can suffer a variety of disorders caused by injury, lack of hygiene, improperly fitting shoes, poor circulation, or disease. Toenail woes include bruises, fungal infections, discoloration, brittleness, and deformity. Seniors, who often neglect their feet because they can't reach them, have arthritis, or lack the hand strength to cut increasingly tough nails, are particularly prone to toenail issues. Overgrown toenails, thick calluses, and cracked, dry heels are often the result.

The Benefits of Barefoot Walking

Feet play an important role in proprioception, which is the gathering of information necessary for awareness of balance, movement, and your position in space. Bare feet touching the ground can relay much more information to the brain than feet encased in shoes. Over time, the constant shielding of feet can lead to a loss of normal nerve response and even painful hypersensitivity.

Stimulating the feet by walking barefoot sends large amounts of data to the brain and helps keep it active and sharp, plus it allows feet to relax, expand, become stronger, and develop better mechanics. If you rarely go barefoot, try spending even just 10 to 15 minutes a day barefoot, preferably outdoors. Choose a safe, textured surface, such as mown grass, soft dirt or sand, or a smooth stone ledge. Wading in a brook or the ocean is great for your feet, too.

Many folks notice that as they spend more time barefoot, they feel

PARTS OF THE TOENAIL

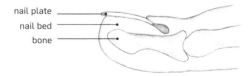

nail plate

nail bed

bone

Fun Foot Test

Let's see just how coordinated your feet are with this simple test.

1. Sit in a straight-backed chair, facing straight ahead, with your feet flat on the floor.

2. Lift your right foot off the ground a few inches (there's no need to point your toes).

3. Start drawing a clockwise circle with your foot. At the same time, write the number 6 in the air with your right hand, repeatedly.

You'll soon see that your right foot follows suit and reverses to counterclockwise motion. Neurological pathways will not allow your foot to move in a different direction than your hand, no matter how hard you try. And believe me, I keep trying!

less anxious and sleep better. Often they have improved circulation in the feet and legs, better clarity of thought, enhanced immunity and vitality, and a decrease in overall inflammation. They feel refreshed, calm, grounded yet energized, and fully alive. Being barefoot feels great once your tender soles get used to the new sensations!

Though I encourage daily barefoot walking (and spend as much time barefoot myself as I can), do be careful. You should not go from regularly wearing shoes, especially ill-fitting ones (and that includes overly padded running/walking shoes with elevated heels and tapered toes), to going straight-up barefoot for any length of time—your feet and lower legs will probably scream! Feet that have been caged for years in typical modern shoes will not function properly, especially on uneven surfaces.

Bare your soles slowly, for a few minutes each day, and work up to more extended time. Weak foot and calf muscles need to be conditioned and strengthened and the bottoms of your feet need to be toughened a bit before you venture forth for any length of time with barefoot confidence. Be careful where you plant your tootsies, and inspect your feet when you return indoors.

Be aware that some folks simply cannot walk barefoot, whether it's because of injury, a foot deformity of some type, or a lack of natural padding on the soles. Diabetics and those suffering from neuropathy in their feet may not realize when their feet suffer tissue damage and should not go barefoot outdoors unless the area is guaranteed to be free of sharp objects, prickly plants, and biting insects.

If it's difficult for you to find safe natural surfaces for barefoot walking, then walk barefoot in your home or on carpeted surfaces as much as you can. Your feet will still become stronger, though you will not experience the energizing, grounding, full-body health benefits of sauntering on the actual earth.

And if walking barefoot on any surface isn't in the best interest of your feet or your body for medical reasons, then you can at least do daily foot exercises; see Chapter 2.

The Shoes You Choose

The shoes you wear have a huge impact on your foot function and therefore your whole body's function. Delving into all the pros and cons of every style of shoe available would fill an entire book, but suffice it to say, most of them are not good for your feet! In fact, the majority of foot problems can be attributed to ill-fitting footwear.

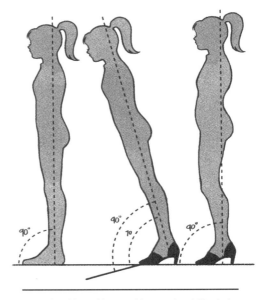

Your shoulders, hips, and knees should be balanced over your ankles for proper posture, as shown on the left. Wearing high heels throws your whole body out of alignment.

Most shoes—for work, athletics, or fashion—are designed not with natural foot function and health in mind, but for pleasure, popularity, and profit. Shoes that are too cushioned or overly supportive, shoes with tight toes and high heels, and shoes that just don't fit properly have spawned an epidemic of foot dysfunctions and deformities.

But it's not just the feet that suffer. Your feet are the foundation of your body, and when they can't move naturally and freely, the rest of the body is negatively impacted. Over time, ill-fitting shoes can cause any of the following:

- Cramps and fatigue in the toes, feet, and legs
- Ongoing pain in the toes, balls of the feet, and heels
- Corns and calluses
- Poor circulation in the feet and lower legs
- Weak arches that don't provide adequate support
- Weak, sore ankles
- Painful, stiff knees, hips, back, and shoulders
- Contraction and other deformities of the toes
- Bunions
- Stress fractures of the foot

When your feet hurt, so do you! Furthermore, these foot problems can lead to issues with balance, as well as headaches, irritability, nervous exhaustion, and general fatigue.

FOOT NOTE

If you must wear fashionable shoes that coerce your feet into unnatural shapes, think of them as dessert. Too much dessert and, well, you know what happens: The body changes shape, and not in a good way. Wear your "fancy" shoes only for special occasions, not all day, every day.

How to Shop for Shoes

Buy the most health-promoting shoes that your feet and your budget can handle. If you must have arch support, lots of stability, and plenty of cushion, that's fine for now. As your feet grow stronger and more flexible—and they will if you wear better shoes and do the exercises outlined in Chapter 2—you can transition to shoes that do a better job of supporting foot health and functionality. You'll eventually discover that your feet will bark in protest if forced back into most modern shoe styles.

Whether your feet are already in great condition or you're working to restore their strength, flexibility, and natural shape, let the suggestions on the following page be your guide for shoe shopping. (See Resources on page 126 for suggested shoe brands that promote healthy feet.)

> *And forget not that the earth delights to feel your bare feet and the winds long to play with your hair.*
>
> —Khalil Gibran, *The Prophet*

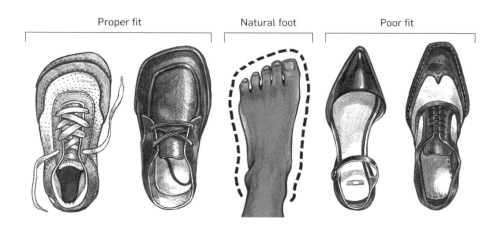

Proper fit   Natural foot   Poor fit

A wide toe box gives your toes room to move. Pointed shoes cramp your toes and restrict natural movement.

PLANNING AHEAD

▶ Feet tend to swell as the day goes by, so buy shoes in the afternoon or at the end of your work cycle when possible.

▶ Bring the type of hosiery that you intend to wear with the style of shoe you are buying.

▶ If you wear orthotics or other special insoles, bring them with you. You'll need a roomier shoe to allow for proper fit and function.

CHOOSING THE RIGHT SHOES

▶ Ideally, shoes should be shaped like normal human feet, not even moderately tapered, and certainly not pointy like elf shoes.

▶ Breathability is key for avoiding soggy, smelly feet and a premature breakdown of shoe materials. Warm, damp feet also encourage the proliferation of foot/toenail fungus. Somewhat porous materials such as leather, polyester or nylon mesh, wool, hemp, bamboo, linen, cork, jute, and cotton allow some of the heat and steam generated inside the shoe to escape.

▶ Shoes should have a flat sole or minimal heel (not more than ½ inch), relatively flexible soles, and no toe spring (an upward-curving toe area). They should bend easily at the ball of the foot, with enough cushioning to be comfortable but not so much that they feel squishy. The uppers should be flexible, too. The toe box should be wide at the forefoot to allow plenty of wiggle room.

▶ Removable insoles give room for orthotics if you have them or can be easily replaced with a different material or thickness if you want.

TRYING SHOES ON

▶ Your feet change in size and shape from year to year, so have them measured while you're standing, not sitting, every time you buy shoes.

▶ Try on both shoes, not just one. Most people have one foot that's slightly larger than the other. Buy shoes that accommodate the longest and widest foot.

- A properly fitting pair of shoes should feel good from the get-go. If they're tight when you try them on, don't expect them to stretch after you've worn them for a while. It's more likely that your feet will accommodate the shoes rather than the other way around.

- Walk around in the store as much as possible before purchasing. Feet expand when walking, so the shoes need to allow for movement. Make sure there is adequate space (approximately a finger's width) between your longest toe and the end of each shoe.

- The heel should be snug and firm enough that it doesn't slip when you walk.

FOOT NOTE

The shoes you wear either undermine or promote healthy feet. You can have shoe-shaped feet or wear feet-shaped shoes—it's your choice!

A Note about Safety Shoes

Physically demanding, high-risk jobs, such as those in construction, agriculture, and many other fields, often require special safety shoes. Usually this type of footwear is constructed of heavy-duty materials and has thick soles and often steel toes.

Of course you need to protect your feet, but these shoes tend to be quite stiff, especially upon purchase. When you buy a pair, make sure they truly fit, are super comfortable, provide the support you need, and don't bind or pinch anywhere.

Quality safety shoes don't come cheap, but neither do medical care and unemployment resulting from a disfigured foot. Don't try to pinch pennies when purchasing protective shoes. Buy the best pair you can afford.

Foot Care Basics

It's a fact: The better you care for your two precious feet, the better the health and quality of life you will be able to enjoy throughout your years. Just follow these simple guidelines for happy feet.

DAILY

▸ Wash your feet, getting between the toes and under the nails. Dry them completely.

▸ Apply foot powder to help absorb perspiration and minimize odor.

▸ Change your socks or hose.

▸ Do a few stretching and strengthening exercises (see Chapter 2).

▸ Wear flat, natural-shaped shoes that encourage healthy, functional feet.

▸ Make sure your shoes are dry, which keeps your feet healthier and makes shoes last longer. If necessary, alternate between pairs of shoes to allow them to completely dry out.

▸ Walk, walk, walk. It strengthens your feet and legs and improves balance and circulation.

▸ Spend some time going barefoot so your feet can breathe and relax, unfettered from the confines of shoes.

WEEKLY OR BIWEEKLY

▸ Inspect your feet for blisters, corns, calluses, swelling, or other problems and treat accordingly. An ounce of prevention is worth a pound of cure, as the saying goes.

▸ Use a quality salt or sugar scrub on your feet and ankles to exfoliate any dead skin buildup, leaving feet smooth and silky. (I recommend Sweet Feet Sugary Foot Scrub, page 70, or Peppermint Salt Glo, page 71.) File or pare down any calluses or corns.

▸ Give yourself a weekly "feet treat." Massage your feet with warmed coconut (fractionated or virgin), jojoba, extra-virgin olive, castor, or almond oil mixed with a couple drops of lavender, peppermint, sweet orange, frankincense, or eucalyptus essential oil. Better yet, ask a friend or family member to rub them for you! Then return the favor. (**Caution:** Avoid using peppermint or eucalyptus essential oils if pregnant or breastfeeding.)

MONTHLY

► Cut your toenails straight across to help avoid ingrown toenails. Afterward, smooth the nail edges with an emery board or file.

► Indulge in a professional pedicure if possible. It feels great and does wonders for your feet. Pedicures are especially recommended for seniors who have difficulty performing routine foot maintenance.

► Make an appointment with a foot reflexologist. Reflexology works through the nervous system to reduce body stress and improve circulation throughout the entire body, plus it helps relieve tension, tightness, and achiness in feet.

I would be remiss if I didn't add this final note about overall foot health: Being overweight increases pressure on the small bones and joints of the feet and exacerbates the risk of damage. I know it's easy to say and hard to do, but losing even a few pounds can help reduce the stress on your feet.

> *You have brains in your head.*
> *You have feet in your shoes.*
> *You can steer yourself*
> *any direction you choose.*
>
> —Dr. Seuss, *Oh, the Places You'll Go!*

FOOT NOTE
Most people have one foot larger than the other; it's rare for both feet to be exactly the same length and width.

2 FOOT FITNESS

Stretching and Strengthening

We all arrive in this world buck naked and barefoot, with a wide forefoot and soft, smooth toes that wiggle freely. In a world devoid of pavement, rocky ground, corporate dress codes, or fashion trends, you could go through life shoeless and carefree, or at the very most in loose sandals in summer and warm, comfy moccasins in winter. But, alas, many of us neither live in such a place nor want to give up our stylish shoes.

Many people experience foot and ankle pain at some point in their lives, whether related to footwear habits or other reasons. For the majority of us, specific exercises for the feet can strengthen and stretch the muscles; relieve cramping and strain in the arches; ease heel pain; reduce the discomfort of hammertoes, bunions, and pinched toes; and relieve general achiness. Consistent exercise will help counter some, though definitely not all, of the negative effects of abusive footwear.

Your feet, just like the rest of your body, need to be toned and stretched in their natural, unbound state. You wear comfortable, unrestrictive clothes when you work out, right? Similarly, avoid constrictive shoes for these stretching and strengthening foot exercises. Go barefoot, or at least slip off your shoes. Do keep in mind, though, that even daily foot exercises will be of minimal benefit if you continue to wear ill-fitting shoes that restrict movement and force your feet into an unnatural shape.

Exercises for Healthy Feet

Regularly exercising and stretching the feet and ankles can help ensure that muscles, ligaments, tendons, and fascia (a weblike connective tissue that weaves and wraps itself through and around virtually everything in the body) are providing the best support and that circulation is strong. These exercises also help improve range of motion in the feet, keeping you active for as long as possible.

FOOT NOTE
The average pair of feet spends 16 hours a day encased in shoes. Try to give your tootsies at least a few unfettered hours a day, and not just when you're in bed. Going barefoot around your home is one way to let them be free.

Your Feet Are Your Foundation

Just as the foundation of a house supports the frame above it and enables the windows and doors to function with ease and floors to remain level, so your feet are designed to support your entire body, promoting balance and comfortable movement. If the foundation of a house becomes unstable, the house will begin to tilt and creak. The same holds true for your body.

If your feet—or even just one of them—become structurally compromised or chronically achy/painful, weak, cramped, or tight, this discomfort will invariably, over time, lead to misalignment of your body, increasing the likelihood of ankle, knee, hip, back, and shoulder problems, gait alteration, and difficulty walking. The dis-ease in your feet will be reflected as dis-ease in your body. The health of your entire body depends on a solid foundation, so keep your feet strong, flexible, agile, and healthy!

Most of these foot, ankle, and toe exercises are relatively simple in concept, but some may prove challenging, especially the Independent Toe Lifts (page 20) and Rocking Horse (page 28). Several of them can be performed any time you feel the need to stretch and release tension. If you can't discreetly slip off your shoes during the day, then perform the exercises when you get home from work or finish your daily errands.

Take off your shoes and take a few minutes to relax and unwind. Try sipping a cup of soothing herbal tea, hot or cold, while you do your exercises, to help you really focus on the moment.

If you experience uncomfortable cramping or deep foot fatigue while performing any exercise, it usually means that your muscles are weak and/or your feet are inflexible and need conditioning. Do fewer repetitions at first, but keep at it. It's what you do on a daily basis that produces long-term results.

Foot Roller Massage

Foot rollers are both stimulating and relaxing to the feet. They've been around for decades and come in all shapes and sizes, from single to double or triple rollers. They can be made of wood, soft rubber with raised nubs, hard plastic, smooth metal, or even Himalayan salt.

Some are handheld, but most are designed to be placed on the floor. I particularly like the ones with raised ridges extending from one end to the other. If you don't have a foot roller, you can use a wooden rolling pin.

This exercise relieves fatigue and muscle cramping, especially in your arches, and delivers relief to tight muscles and the plantar fascia ligament. Rolling your soles is a great way to begin exercising your feet.

Sit up straight in a chair with your feet flat on the floor. (Or, if you have good balance or something to hold on to, you can perform this exercise while standing.)

Place the foot roller on the floor and, while bearing down comfortably, roll the entire length of your foot, from the base of your toes to your heel, back and forth over the roller.

Continue rolling for at least 5 minutes, then switch to the other foot.

ALTERNATIVE A frozen water bottle makes a soothing foot roller when your feet are hot, achy, and swollen.

VARIATION If you have sensitive feet (or don't have a foot roller), you can use a tennis ball or other relatively firm, small ball to massage your soles.

Place your foot on the ball and roll it the length of your foot, pressing down as hard as is comfortable. You should feel a nice release of tension. Continue for 5 minutes, then repeat with your other foot.

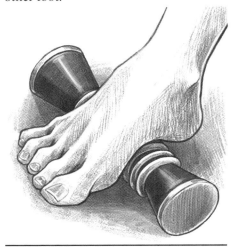

Using a foot roller

17

WHAT YOU NEED

4	tablespoons dried yarrow, sage, or peppermint, or 8 tablespoons chopped fresh herbs (optional)
	Large tea ball, reusable tea bag, or square of muslin (if you are using herbs)
½	cup sea salt, baking soda, or Epsom salts
5	drops rosemary or eucalyptus essential oil
3	drops grapefruit, lavender, or peppermint essential oil
	Foot-soaking basin
2	bath towels
40–60	medium to large marbles (use large marbles if you have long toes)

FOOT REFRESHER AND REVITALIZER

This combined exercise and foot soak is designed to relax tired, aching feet, relieve toe cramps, and strengthen the muscles that support the arches, while also reducing stress on the plantar fascia ligament. It makes stinky dogs smell better, too! The herbs are optional but definitely add refreshing and deodorizing benefits.

1 If you are using the herbs, put them in a tea ball or tea bag or tie them up in a square of muslin (or you may add them in loose form). Bring 2 cups of water to a boil in a small pot and then remove from the heat. Add the herbs, cover, and let steep for 15 minutes. Remove or strain the herbs and discard them.

2 Add the sea salt, baking soda, or Epsom salts and the essential oils to the basin and pour the hot tea over them. Fill the tub with warm tap water to make the soaking water as hot as you find comfortable.

3 Place the tub on a bath towel on the floor in front of a comfortable chair, then add the marbles. Place your feet in the tub and roll them around on the marbles. Pick up and release the marbles with your toes, grasping the marbles tightly, squeezing your toes, then releasing. Do this for 10 to 15 minutes. Then dry your feet roughly with a fresh towel.

When you're done, slather your feet with a thick moisturizer or conditioning oil (try the Comfrey Foot Massage Oil, page 19), and then put on socks to help your chosen product sink in.

Note: Safe for folks 6 years of age and older; if pregnant or breastfeeding, omit the rosemary, eucalyptus, and peppermint essential oils and use 8 drops total of grapefruit and lavender essential oils

WHAT YOU NEED

1–2 teaspoons comfrey-infused oil

2–4 drops cedarwood, lavender, and/ or sweet orange essential oil

COMFREY FOOT MASSAGE OIL

After soaking and exercising your feet, use this therapeutic herbal oil to relax even further while also conditioning rough skin. Comfrey-infused oil (available from many natural foods stores and herbal companies) is particularly recommended if your feet are itchy, irritated, frequently achy, or inflamed. This is a lovely treatment right before bedtime.

Mix all the ingredients thoroughly in a very small bowl. Massage the oil into your feet and calves using a firm, strong hand, applying pressure as needed to alleviate fatigue and tension.

When you're done, put on a pair of socks to help the oil sink in.

TO MAKE A LARGER QUANTITY, combine ¼ cup of comfrey-infused oil with 8 drops each of the essential oil(s) you're using in a 2-ounce dark glass bottle with a dropper top. Screw the top on the bottle and shake vigorously for 2 minutes to blend.

Label and date the bottle and set it in a cool, dark location for 24 hours so that the oils can synergize. Store at room temperature, away from heat and light; use within 1 year. Shake well before each use.

Note: Safe for folks over 12 years of age; for children aged 6–11, use only 2 drops of essential oil; if pregnant or breastfeeding, avoid cedarwood essential oil

Point and Flex

This is a great exercise to stretch and relax just about everything from your knees down. It's wonderful if you suffer from plantar fasciitis or cramping and tightness in the toes, feet, and calves.

Position yourself in one of two ways: sitting on the floor, legs stretched out in front of you and palms on the floor at your sides, or seated in a chair with both legs extended in front of you.

Point your feet and toes away from you (like a ballerina) as hard as you can and hold for 5 seconds. Then flex your feet, pulling your toes toward your shins as hard as you can, and hold for 5 seconds. Repeat 10 times.

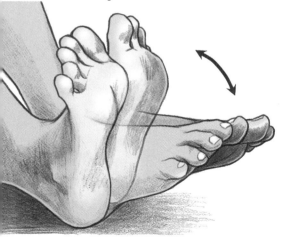

Independent Toe Lifts

The 10 small intrinsic muscles in the sole of each foot work together to stabilize the arches and individually to control the movement of your toes. Your hands have the same type of muscles, and just as your fingers can move individually, so should your toes. Is that possible? Yes!

Why do you need to do this exercise? It's not like you're going to be writing with your toes, but good flexibility, dexterity, strength, and circulation make for a healthy foot. Mastering the independent movement of each toe takes a lot of practice, and not everyone can do it, even after working at it for months. Your feet will probably feel fatigued at first, but do the best you can, and you just might be pleasantly surprised by what your toes can do!

You can either sit or stand for this exercise. Just make sure you are comfortable and balanced. If you're standing, steady yourself by holding on to the back of a chair or wall, if needed.

Aim your feet straight ahead, keeping them flat on the floor. Press your big toes into the ground and lift the other four toes as high as you can. Your feet might feel confused and uncoordinated;

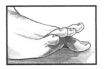

that's okay. Just focus on pressing your big toe downward and slightly away from the other toes. Hold for 5 seconds, then relax. Repeat five times for each foot.

Now do the reverse, pressing your four small toes into the ground while

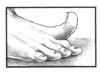

lifting your big toe as high as you can. Hold for 5 seconds, then relax. Repeat five times for each foot.

Things get more advanced when you try to raise each toe individually. Make sure to keep your feet flat on the floor and pointed straight ahead. Do not roll your ankles in either direction in an attempt to raise your toes.

Begin by raising your big toes as high as you can, then lower them. Repeat five times. Next, try to raise just your second toes, then lower them. Repeat five times. Continue with the remaining toes.

Heel-to-Toe Stress Releaser

This sequential exercise will help stretch and strengthen all parts of your feet and toes. You will feel this workout in your feet—I guarantee it!

Sit up straight in a chair with your feet flat on the floor.

1. Raise your heels. Stop when only the balls of your feet and toes remain on the floor—the same position your feet would be in if you were wearing very high heels. Hold this position for 5 seconds, then lower your heels to the floor.

2. Raise just your toes. Hold for 5 seconds and then release them.

3. Flex your feet, pulling your toes toward your shins. Keep your heels on the floor. Hold for 5 seconds and then release.

4. Place your feet flat on the floor. Raise your heels and point your toes, so that only the tips of your big toe and second toe are touching the floor— as if you were a ballerina standing in toe shoes. You should feel your calves contracting. Hold for 5 seconds and then release.

5. Curl all your toes under and squeeze hard. Hold for 5 seconds and then release.

Repeat the entire sequence 10 times, then shake your feet out and do a few ankle rotations in each direction.

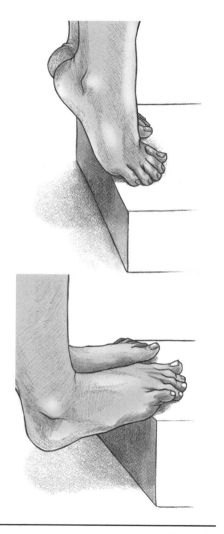

Lower and raise your heels slowly, holding each position for 5 seconds.

Heel Raises

This is a good exercise if you regularly wear high heels or any style of shoe that has even a 1-inch heel rise (this includes many running and walking shoes, men's dress shoes, construction boots, and so-called "flats"). Heel raises strengthen your ankle, improve your balance, stretch the Achilles tendon and plantar fascia, and provide overall foot conditioning.

This exercise is best performed on a step or exercise bench, though any similar structure—a length of 6×6 lumber, landscape timber, or even a concrete curb—will work. Whatever you use, make sure it's well braced and won't tip or roll over.

Stand on the step with the balls of your feet at the edge, your heels hanging off, and your toes pointing straight ahead. Lower your heels *slowly* as far as they will comfortably go (you should feel a good stretch in the back of your calves) and maintain this position for 5 seconds.

Then slowly rise up on your toes as high as you can comfortably go, contracting your calf muscles, and hold this position for 5 seconds. Repeat the exercise 15 to 20 times.

Runner's Stretch

This exercise is recommended for anyone who regularly wears shoes with a 1-inch or higher heel. It's good for runners or walkers as a warm-up stretch for their lower leg muscles, and it stretches the plantar fascia and Achilles tendon, making it useful for relieving heel pain and plantar fasciitis.

The runner's stretch is somewhat like doing a modified push-up against a wall. Stand a bit more than arm's length from a wall.

With your right foot only, step forward about halfway toward the wall. Place your palms against the wall, keeping your left leg straight and both heels flat on the floor. You should feel the back of your left calf and the entire sole of your foot stretching.

Hold this position for at least 10 seconds. Return to the starting position, relax, and repeat 10 to 20 times. Switch legs and repeat.

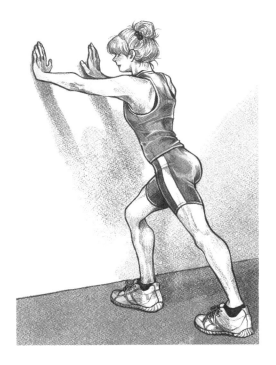

Ankle Rotations

This simple exercise helps relieve stiffness and tension and improve circulation in the ankle joint and adjacent areas of the foot and calf. I especially recommend it if you suffer from arthritic ankles and foot cramps. It feels great performed at the end of a long day on your feet or after long periods of sitting.

Sit up straight in a chair with your feet flat on the floor. Extend your legs comfortably out in front of you and simply draw circles with your feet, 20 times each, first clockwise, then counterclockwise. If it's easier, you can do this with one foot at a time.

Rubber Band Big Toe Stretches

This exercise is helpful if you suffer from bunions or cramping in the medial longitudinal arch (see page 3), which can often result from regularly wearing any shoe styles with a tapered toe box or high heels, or shoes that are too short for your feet. You'll need a thick rubber band 1½ to 2 inches in diameter; the kind used to bundle broccoli stalks or asparagus spears would work.

Position yourself in one of two ways: sitting on the floor, legs stretched out in front of you and palms on the floor at your sides or behind you, or seated in a chair with your feet flat on the floor.

Bring your feet together and place the rubber band around your big toes. Keeping your heels together, pull your toes away from each other, making a narrow V with your feet.

Hold for 5 to 10 seconds, then relax. Repeat 10 to 20 times. If this hurts, or if you have arthritis or bunions, do only as many repetitions as you can and gradually increase as your toes gain strength.

Perform this exercise three times per day (and stop wearing shoes that squinch your toes together!).

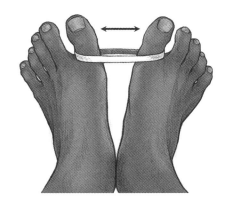

Draw the Alphabet

This fun exercise aims to loosen and relax all parts of the feet and ankles while promoting flexibility. It's especially helpful if you suffer from plantar fasciitis or everyday stiffness and discomfort. Do it at the end of the day after you've been on your feet for hours and your dogs are barking.

While sitting in warm bathwater, or while soaking your feet in a warm footbath, slowly draw the alphabet with your feet by using your big toe as the tip of the "pencil." Repeat the entire alphabet twice with each foot. Your feet will say "Ahhh . . ."

Toe Spread

Lots of folks can't spread their toes at all, but your toes, like your fingers, are meant to flex in all directions. This exercise may take lots of consistent practice to master. It is especially recommended for those suffering from bunions, toe cramps, neuromas, metatarsalgia (pain in the ball of the foot), and arch and shin pain. Over time, it will help create a wider base of support in the forefoot, align toes, improve balance and stability, strengthen muscles throughout the foot and lower leg, and help restore foot function.

Sit in a comfortable chair with just your heels resting on the floor. Curl your toes tightly downward for 5 seconds, then lift your toes and spread them as far apart as they will go, like you would spread your fingers.

Hold this position for 10 seconds. Really focus on awakening your "brain to foot" communication. Release and relax. Repeat the exercise five times, three times per day.

TO IMPROVE TOE SPREAD. For toes that are particularly tight, I suggest wearing toe separators such as Correct Toes or YogaToes. Follow the directions for use on the package, and know that the secret to success with these types of products is consistency. Realigning the bones of your feet takes time, and depending on how tightly your toes are compressed, you may be able to wear them for only 15 minutes at a time without undue pain. Keep at it and your feet will improve, I promise!

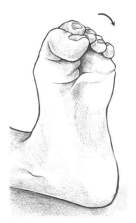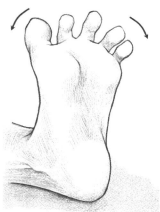

Shake Hands with Your Feet

Though this exercise has a humorous name, it provides a serious stretch for your forefoot and toes and feels especially good after you've been on your feet all day—whether shod or barefoot. If your toes are tight and relatively immobile, you may have a difficult time sliding your fingers between them, but keep practicing every single day. Your toes didn't get into their current state overnight, so don't expect flexibility miracles.

People with short or chubby toes and/or large fingers may not be able to perform this exercise. Don't dismay. Practice some of the other toe exercises, such as the Toe Spread (page 25) or Independent Toe Lifts (page 20). Also, this one may not be to your liking if you have very sensitive toes or super-ticklish feet.

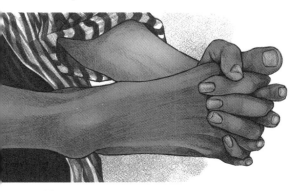

Sit up straight in a chair, in a comfortable position. Cross your left leg over your right knee, resting your ankle on top of your knee so that you can easily reach your toes with your right hand.

Slowly slide your fingers in between your toes from the bottom of your foot. Work your fingers in as far as they will go without causing pain—though a little discomfort is to be expected at first.

Let your fingers rest there for a minute or two, if possible, and then slide them back out. Even if you can only get just the tips of your fingers between your toes, you are giving the surrounding muscles more of a stretch than they've had in a long while.

If your toes are nimble and you can insert your fingers all the way down to their base, wrap your thumb around the outside of your big toe and close your fingers, as if you were "shaking hands" with your toes. With your hands in this position, move your forefoot back and forth and also in circular motions so that it feels nice and loose. Do this for 1 to 2 minutes.

Switch legs and repeat on the other foot. Do this exercise two or three times per day.

ALTERNATIVE If you can't easily cross your legs and reach your toes, ask a friend, family member, foot reflexologist, or massage therapist for help.

Towel Pick-Up

If you suffer from achy feet, hammertoes, metatarsalgia (pain in the ball of the foot), stiff ankles, pain in the arches, or toe cramps, this exercise is for you. It also improves dexterity in the toes.

Place a small, thin bath towel or large hand towel on the floor in front of a chair. Leave it bunched up and slightly wrinkled so it is easier to grasp.

Sitting in the chair, grip the towel with your toes, using both feet. Lift and straighten your legs out in front of you. Hold for 10 seconds, then release the towel. Repeat 10 times.

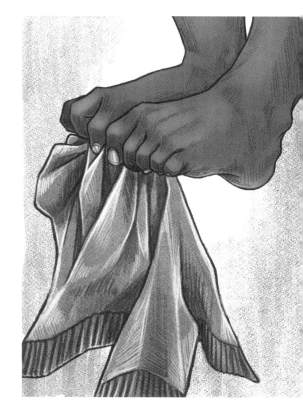

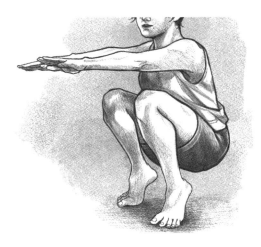

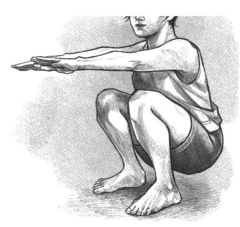

Rocking Horse

This advanced movement improves your balance, conditions your entire lower body, and helps stretch and strengthen all the muscles in your feet. Your Achilles tendon gets a nice workout, too. You need to be limber, strong, balanced, and agile for this exercise, but it's worth trying even if you're not. The more you do it, the easier it will become.

I like to do this exercise while doing the "breaststroke" in the air. As I squat down on my toes, I extend my arms out to the sides for balance. Then, as I roll back, I slowly bring my arms forward until they are fully extended in front of me. As I return to my tiptoes, I bring my arms back out to the sides. After 10 to 15 repetitions, I feel as if I've had a mini workout in my lower body.

Stand with your feet about shoulder width apart, with one hand holding on to a chair, doorway frame, or deck post to steady yourself, if necessary. Now, squat all the way down until you are resting on your tiptoes.

Slowly roll back until you are resting flat on your feet, hold for 5 seconds, then slowly roll forward again until you are back on your tiptoes. Work up to 10 repetitions.

Commonsense caution: If you have hip, knee, or ankle replacements, or if you have had foot, ankle, or lower leg surgery involving bone fusions, insertion of screws, or metal plates, please check with your orthopedic surgeon prior to performing this exercise, as it may be contraindicated.

Get Moving!

Walking is one of the best whole-body exercises. Walking at a brisk pace with your arms pumping provides cardiovascular benefits, improves circulation, burns calories, and strengthens the body from the feet up by engaging the muscles in your legs, buttocks, lower back, and abdomen. If your feet and legs tend to swell or you suffer from Raynaud's disease or varicose veins, walking will help improve those issues by boosting vital circulation to the extremities.

Make sure to wear walking or running shoes that are super comfortable, have a wide forefoot so your toes can wiggle, and are flexible in the sole, so that your feet can propel you forward like they are designed to do. Avoid athletic shoes that are so heavily padded and stiff that you can't really feel the terrain you are walking on.

Alternatively, if you have healthy, strong feet and walking barefoot for at least 20 minutes doesn't cause undue discomfort, then by all means find a park, well-groomed trail, or sandy beach on which to take your walk sans shoes.

After a walk, do a few foot exercises. Try to get into the habit of walking for health at least four or five times per week, and work up to 30 or 45 minutes each session.

Commonsense caution: If you're out of shape or physically not able to do brisk walking, begin by taking short, slow walks within your comfort zone, adding more time as you're able. Do the best you can. See your healthcare provider if you have health concerns.

Keep your feet on the ground and keep reaching for the stars.

—Casey Kasem, creator of American Top 40

3

FOOT MASSAGE

to Relax and Revive

The therapeutic use of massage (the word comes from the Arabic *massa*, meaning "to stroke") dates back thousands of years and is well documented in writing and images from China, Egypt, Japan, and elsewhere. The Greek physician Hippocrates was a proponent, writing, "The physician must be experienced in many things, but most assuredly in rubbing."

The benefits of foot massage are many: It helps reduce stress and anxiety, soothe the nervous system, and boost circulation (blood, lymph, energy flow) while minimizing any swelling.

It relieves muscle soreness, tension, knots, and joint pain in all parts of the feet, which relaxes your entire body and improves sleep quality (especially if performed before bedtime). And if you also apply a soothing balm, oil, or lotion, it will dramatically soften your skin.

Although not as fulfilling as having your feet massaged by someone else, self-massage lets you de-stress and care for yourself by pampering your feet as you see fit. And while being on the receiving end of a massage is clearly the best position, giving a friend or loved one a foot massage is soothing and calming for you, too. It can even promote a reduction in your blood pressure. It's a caring, nurturing, and bonding experience to share with another person.

If you've been on your feet all day, your nerves are frayed, and your energy tank is running on empty, an aromatherapy foot massage will soothe your spirits, put the spring back in your step, and soften your feet. After all, what's good for the body is good for the "sole"!

Swollen Feet?

Feet and ankles can swell from sitting too long in one position (taking a long flight or drive, sitting at your desk, watching a movie, et cetera) or if you've been on your feet all day. Elevate your legs to reduce swelling. Lie down or sit in a recliner and lift your legs above your heart, resting them on a pillow, if possible. Do this for at least 20 minutes. Engaging a friend or family member to give you a foot and lower leg massage for about 10 minutes (with the promise to reciprocate) will get circulation moving and relax tension. You'll feel *sooo* much better afterward.

Techniques of Foot Massage

These illustrations depict some standard foot relaxation techniques that a licensed nail technician, massage therapist, or foot reflexologist might perform on a client. If you do not have a willing partner to give you a massage, never fear. These techniques are easily adjusted for self-massage.

Have the person receiving the foot massage sit in a recliner or lounge chair with their feet elevated so that their body is fully relaxed. Foot massage feels particularly great when the whole body is at ease. Make sure that you can comfortably reach their feet from your own seat, without having to lean or hunch over.

If you're going solo, find a comfortable chair, preferably one with padded arms and a footrest, such as a recliner or a small loveseat with an ottoman. Sit back and cross one leg over the other, with the sole facing you and the other leg extended.

A FEW TIPS

▸ When using massage oil or lotion, grab a towel or two to protect furniture and clothing.

▸ Rub your hands together vigorously to warm them before beginning the massage.

▸ Perform any massage technique on both feet (no playing favorites, even if one foot is achier than the other).

▸ Complete all the steps on one foot before moving to the other.

Step 1: Stroke

Gentle stroking, using light to moderate pressure, stimulates circulation and relaxes and warms the lower leg and foot muscles. Start by stroking and gently squeezing your partner's calf from just below the back of the knee to just above the ankle. Use alternating hands to do this.

Next, hold your partner's foot in your hands, with your fingers supporting the sole and thumbs on top. Make long, slow, firm stroking motions with your thumbs, starting at the base of the toes and gliding away from you to the ankle; then glide back to where you began using a lighter stroke. Cover the entire top surface of the foot. Repeat three to five times.

Next, place your hands on either side of the foot, with your thumbs on the sole and fingers on top. Perform back and forth horizontal strokes or thumb slides, beginning at the ball of the foot and moving down over the arches to the base of the heel, then reverse and work your thumbs back to the ball of the foot. Your strokes should be firm, with moderate pressure. Repeat three to five times.

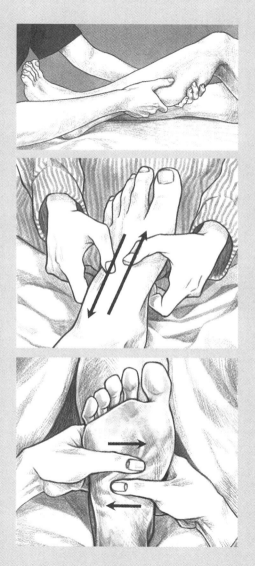

Step 2: Ankle Rotations

This technique loosens the ankle joints and relaxes the feet. Cup one hand under your partner's heel, behind the ankle, to brace the foot and leg.

Grasp the foot with your other hand, placing your thumb on the ball of the foot and four fingers on top of the foot, covering the metatarsals (the forefoot area below the toes). The web of your thumb should be wrapped around the lateral (outer) side of the foot, just beneath the base of the little toe.

Slowly rotate the foot at the ankle, 10 times in each direction. With repeated foot massages, any stiffness will begin to recede. This is a particularly good technique for anyone suffering from arthritis.

Step 3: Toe Rotations

Toes, like fingers, are quite sensitive to the touch. This calming massage technique increases flexibility for tight toes. For support, grasp the foot with one hand, placing your thumb on the ball of the foot and four fingers on top of the foot, covering the area below the toes. The web of your thumb should be wrapped around the medial (inner) side of the foot, just beneath the base of the big toe.

With your other hand, grasp the base of the big toe, with your thumb on the bottom and your index and third fingers on top.

Now, gently but firmly lift the joint with a slight upward pull (don't yank) and rotate the toe a few times in each direction. Work your way through all the toes, stabilizing each one at the base.

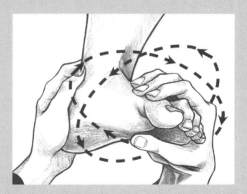

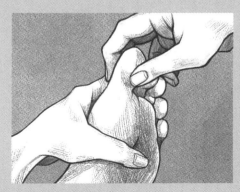

Step 4: Spinal Twist

This foot-wringing technique squeezes out built-up tension, deeply relaxing the muscles and arches. With both hands, grasp the foot from the instep area, on the medial side between the ankle and toes, placing your fingers on top of the foot and your thumbs on the sole. All eight fingers should be touching.

When you're working the left foot, place your left hand just below the ankle joint on top of the foot, and vice versa for your right hand on the right foot. The hand closest to the ankle provides support, while the hand closest to the toes twists slowly and smoothly back and forth as far as possible in each direction.

After several twists, move both hands slightly toward the toes and repeat the twisting action, keeping your fingers touching at all times. The hand closest to the ankle remains stationary, while the hand closest to the toes twists.

Continue this movement (reposition your hands, grip, twist; reposition your hands, grip, twist) until the hand nearest the toes is over the big toe. Make sure you are not twisting both hands at the same time. Repeat three to five times, beginning each time by the ankle.

Why is this called "spinal twist," you ask? If you look at the foot reflexology chart on page 44, you will see that the reflexes that correspond with the human spine are located along the medial edge of the foot. This twisting massage encourages the spinal column and adjacent muscles to relax, promoting a more comfortable back and neck.

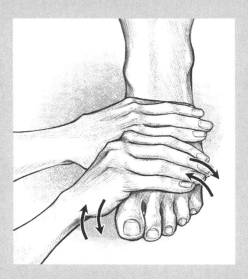

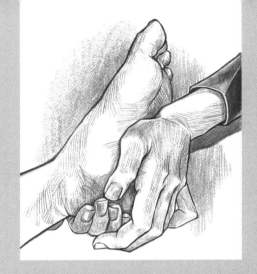

Step 5: Arch Press

To release tension in the plantar fascia and medial longitudinal arch, cup one hand under the heel, behind the ankle, to brace the foot and leg; your fingertips should be on the medial side of the ankle.

Using the heel of your other hand, push moderately hard as you slide along this arch from the ball of the foot down toward the heel and back up again.

Repeat five times. This part of the foot can stand a little extra exertion on your part; just don't apply *too* much pressure.

Step 6: Stroke

Repeat step 1. This is a good way to both begin and end a foot massage.

Foot Massage Elixirs

Foot massage can be performed with or without oils, lotions, or creams. It's easier to grip your own or your partner's foot if it's dry, but a small amount of lubricant makes for easy sliding and gliding over the skin. Don't overdo it, though, or the foot you are working on will be too slippery to hold.

These three recipes are easy to make and leave your paws, as well as your dogs, exceptionally soft, comfortable, and pampered.

Apply the oil or balm before the massage, rubbing it into the skin with firm pressure. Don a pair of socks after the massage to absorb any excess oil and soften the feet.

> *If people bound and gagged the entire body the way they do their feet, none of us would live to the age of twenty.*
>
> —Gordon Inkeles and Murray Todris, *The Art of Sensual Massage*

YIELD

1 treatment

WHAT YOU NEED

1–2 teaspoons almond, extra-virgin olive, fractionated coconut, jojoba, or castor oil

2–4 drops eucalyptus, grapefruit, lemon, and/or peppermint essential oil

FOOT FITNESS MASSAGE OIL

This stimulating, ultrarefreshing, cooling formula helps improve circulation while combating odor.

Mix all the ingredients thoroughly in a very small bowl. Massage the oil into your feet using a firm, strong hand.

TO MAKE A LARGER QUANTITY, combine ¼ cup of base oil with 6 drops each of the essential oil(s) you're using in a 2-ounce dark glass bottle with a dropper top. Screw the top on the bottle and shake vigorously for 2 minutes to blend.

    Label and date the bottle and set it in a cool, dark location for 24 hours so that the oils can synergize. Store at room temperature, away from heat and light; use within 1 year (2 years if you used jojoba oil as your base). Shake well before each use.

Note: Safe for folks 12 years of age and older; for children aged 6–11, use only 2 drops of essential oil; if pregnant or breastfeeding, avoid eucalyptus and peppermint essential oils

"AGONY OF THE FEET" COMFORTING MASSAGE OIL

WHAT YOU NEED

1–2 teaspoons almond, extra-virgin olive, fractionated coconut, jojoba, or castor oil

2 drops ginger essential oil

1 drop Roman chamomile or sweet marjoram essential oil

This is my go-to blend that I use just before bedtime if I've had a particularly tough day, my mind won't shut down, and my feet hurt. It relaxes and warms feet, improves circulation, helps reduce achiness, and gently transports your chaotic mind into a more zenlike state.

Mix all the ingredients thoroughly in a very small bowl. Massage into your feet using a firm, strong hand.

BONUS USE: To help you sleep, apply any leftover oil to your chest and neck, and then cup your hands over your nose and mouth and breathe deeply for 30 seconds.

TO MAKE A LARGER QUANTITY, combine ¼ cup of base oil with 16 drops of ginger essential oil and 8 drops of Roman chamomile or sweet marjoram essential oil in a 2-ounce dark glass bottle with a dropper top. Screw the top on the bottle and shake vigorously for 2 minutes to blend.

Label and date the bottle and set it in a cool, dark location for 24 hours so that the oils can synergize. Store at room temperature, away from heat and light; use within 1 year (2 years if you used jojoba oil as your base). Shake well before each use.

Note: Safe for folks 6 years of age and older

CREAMY COCOA BUTTER FOOT BALM

This thick, pleasantly fragrant balm melts into the skin with nary a trace of greasiness. It conditions and hydrates, leaving feet soft, smooth, and nurtured.

YIELD

4 ounces

WHAT YOU NEED

4 tablespoons almond, extra-virgin olive, or jojoba oil

3–4 tablespoons cocoa butter (depending on the desired thickness)

1 teaspoon vegetable glycerin

400 IU vitamin E oil (in capsules)

24 drops frankincense, lavender, peppermint, and/or sweet orange essential oil (optional)

Dark glass or plastic jars (enough to hold 4 ounces)

1 Combine the base oil, cocoa butter, and glycerin in a small saucepan or double boiler over low heat and warm them until the solids are just melted. Remove from the heat and gently stir with a small spoon for about 1 minute, then allow the mixture to cool for about 5 minutes.

2 Add the vitamin E oil (pierce the capsules and squeeze out the contents) and the essential oil(s), if desired, and blend thoroughly.

3 To incorporate the water-soluble glycerin into the fat-based oil and cocoa butter, set the pan in a shallow ice bath or on top of a flat ice pack. Using a small whisk or spoon, stir at a moderate pace for 4 to 5 minutes, until the product thickens. In the last minute, it will change rapidly and become a light, creamy yellow with the consistency of paste wax. Quickly spoon it into the jars.

Cap, label, and date. Set aside for 24 hours. Store at room temperature, away from heat and light; use within 1 year. The texture of the finished product will depend on the ambient temperature; it softens as it warms.

With this balm, a little goes a long way. I use about ½ teaspoon per foot, or a bit more if I want to massage my lower legs. Scoop out the desired amount and rub it between your hands to soften and warm it, then massage it into your feet.

Note: Safe for folks 6 years of age and older; for children under 6 and those with supersensitive or fragile skin, omit the essential oils; if pregnant or breastfeeding, avoid peppermint essential oil

4

AN INTRODUCTION TO
FOOT
REFLEXOLOGY

Just what is reflexology? According to the Reflexology Association of America, reflexology "maps a reflection of the body predominately on the feet, hands, and outer ears. It uses unique manual techniques to deliver pressure to neural pathways assisting the body to function optimally." It is recognized worldwide by various national health institutions and the public at large as a distinct complementary practice within the holistic health field.

That's the "official" definition. Let me add a bit more detail: The science of reflexology is based on the principle that reflexes in the feet, hands, ears, and face correspond to every organ, gland, structure, and system in the body. By properly pinpointing and working with these reflexes, the reflexologist helps the body create balance.

Reflexology works through the nervous system, and as the practitioner stimulates the energy currents within the body, it is akin to opening a dam to allow a river to flow unimpeded. Reflexology opens the life-giving, flowing river of your body—be it on a physical, energetic, or emotional level—encouraging smooth, harmonious circulation of anything that needs to move, whether that's blood, lymph, energy, nerve impulses, breath, or even stuck emotions and thoughts.

Reflexology can be of significant aid in the reduction of stress, tension, and constriction in the body, conditions that can manifest as constipation, congestion, pain, high blood pressure, rapid heart rate, headache, shortness of breath, and more. When the body is deeply relaxed and its energy is flowing, the conditions for healing are enhanced.

And because reflexology includes manual relaxation techniques, it can soothe the muscles, tendons, fascia, joints, and ligaments in your feet and ankles, too. It often eases swelling and general achiness and encourages more comfortable movement. As I tell my clients, "Better health begins with the sole!"

A Brief History

Reflexology could be described as a transcultural phenomenon, but exactly where and how it all began is somewhat elusive. Many ancient cultures such as the Egyptian, Chinese, Japanese, Babylonian, and others have for thousands of years practiced some type of foot/hand pressure therapy as a mode of preventive and therapeutic medicine.

> *The "sole-ution" to great health and vitality has always been right under our feet! Our feet are too often the most neglected part of our body. This is unfortunate, since they literally carry us through life.*
>
> —Myra Achorn, board-certified reflexologist

The Cherokee people of North America acknowledge the importance of working on the feet in maintaining physical, mental, and spiritual balance. This sacred therapy, practiced for generations within the Cherokee tribes, is often combined with the use of beneficial herbs.

The knowledge of ancient foot reflex therapy (which was often a combination of specific pressure application and therapeutic foot massage) might have been lost to antiquity had it not been for inquiring medical minds of the late nineteenth and early twentieth centuries. William Fitzgerald, an ear, nose, and throat specialist, is widely considered the founder of zone therapy.

Dr. Fitzgerald tested the theories of Austrian physician H. Bressler on his patients and discovered that pressure applied to specific places on the nose, hands, fingers, mouth, throat, tongue, and feet—using ordinary surgical clamps, elastic bands, nasal probes, and aluminum combs—would produce a numbing effect in another area of the body, enabling him to perform some minor surgical procedures with little or no anesthesia.

In 1919 he and his colleague, Dr. Edwin Bowers, wrote *Zone Therapy, or, Curing Pain and Disease*, describing their theory and providing illustration of the ten longitudinal zones of the body. Another physician, Dr. Joseph Shelby Riley, later created drawings of the reflex points on the feet.

Dr. Riley's assistant, Eunice Ingham Stopfel, carried their work even further by mapping out the entire body on the feet and discovering how particular points on the feet correspond with the anatomy and zonal layout of the body. She and her nephew, Dwight Byers, founded the International Institute of Reflexology in the mid-1970s. Because of her tireless and successful efforts, she is often touted as the mother of modern reflexology.

If you're interested in learning more, I highly recommend *Reflexology: Art, Science & History*, by Christine Issel.

The Fundamentals of Reflexology

Ponder this: When your feet hurt, what is the first thing that you do? Remove your shoes and rub the sore spots, right? If you have a backache, you stretch and try to rub between your shoulder blades or lower back. These are instinctive reflexes to try to increase circulation to the area that's hurting or tense and massage out the pain. Frequently it helps.

Reflexology, though, should not be confused with massage, which is the manipulation of the soft tissues of the body using a variety of techniques with varying pressure to improve circulation and reduce muscle and connective tissue tension. A massage session may include the feet but is not typically focused specifically on the feet. Yes, there are similarities in effect, such as deep relaxation, stress reduction, localized pain relief, and improved circulation, but that's where the similarities end.

Zone Theory, Horizontal Guidelines, and Reflex Areas

Since ancient times, healers have employed various hands-on approaches to balance and strengthen the body's energy flow. Many of these methodologies, including acupressure, acupuncture, and shiatsu, agree that this energy flows in meridians or zones (neural pathways) throughout the body. Zone theory is the basis of modern foot reflexology, which uses longitudinal zones as a guideline for organizing relationships or associations between various parts of the body.

There are 10 equal longitudinal zones running the length of the body from the top of the head to the tips of the toes and extending down the arms to the tips of the fingers. Each toe and each finger fall into one zone, with the right big toe, for example, occurring in the same zone as the right thumb, and so on. The 10 zones correspond to the number of fingers and toes and therefore provide a convenient numbering system.

In the neck and head area, the numbered zones intersect. The zones are also considered to pass through the body, so that a zone located on the front of the body is found on the back of the body, and on the top and bottom of the foot. All the organs, glands, structures, and systems lie along one or more of these zones.

If any part of a zone is stressed, the whole zone will be affected through the entire length of the body. When the reflexologist detects sensitivity in a specific part of the foot, they know that it signals something out of balance in that zone somewhere in the body. Similarly, applying direct pressure to any part of a zone will affect the entire zone, not just in the spot or particular reflex point that exhibits sensitivity. This is the basis of zone theory.

In addition to the longitudinal zones, reflexology also utilizes four horizontal guidelines. Their main purpose is to help set the image of the body onto the feet in the proper location and perspective. The guidelines commonly used are the shoulder line, the diaphragm line, the waistline, and the pelvic line.

When you view a reflexology diagram of the feet, you will see that the entire body is charted or mapped out in relation to the zones and guidelines and where specific physical reflex areas are located on the feet. Your feet are a direct reiteration of the body itself, a reflection or mirror image of the body. The right foot reflects the right side of the body, and the left foot reflects the left side of the body.

During every reflexology session, a good practitioner should work all of the zones and reflex areas on both feet to encourage harmonious balance within the body. All of our body systems are interconnected. Our heart, which is part of our circulatory system, does not beat unless our brain, which is part of our nervous system, tells it to. Our skeletal system depends on our digestive system

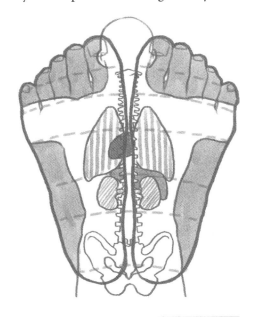

The parts of the feet correspond to the organs and structures of the body.

10 LONGITUDINAL ZONES (5 ON EACH SIDE OF THE BODY)

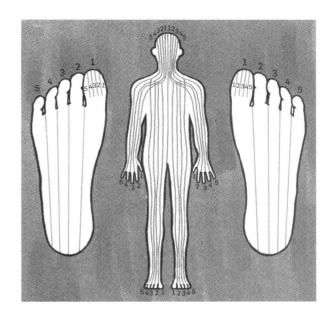

4 HORIZONTAL GUIDELINES

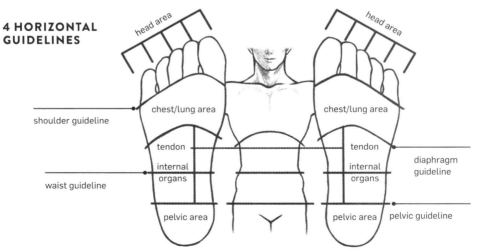

head area

head area

chest/lung area

chest/lung area

shoulder guideline

tendon

tendon

diaphragm guideline

internal organs

internal organs

waist guideline

pelvic area

pelvic area

pelvic guideline

REFLEXOLOGY FOOT MAP

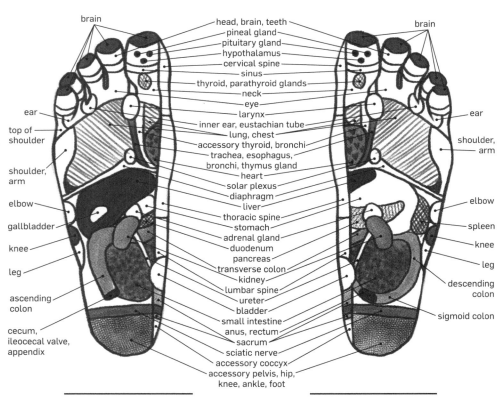

The right foot corresponds to the right side of the body.

The left foot corresponds to the left side of the body.

for its growth and strength. No body part stands alone.

In particular, reflexology can greatly reduce the negative effects of stress and tension. Your feet are extremely receptive to touch and exceptionally responsive to the calming, harmonizing effects of a reflexology session. I've seen it time after time with clients who come feeling unwell, in pain, sad, tense, or depressed and leave in a better, more clarified mood and with improved physical comfort. If you haven't already, I urge you to try this amazingly effective therapy. You'll be hooked and wonder why you never tried it before—because when your feet feel good, so do you.

Key Benefits of Reflexology

Reflexology makes you feel great all over. I guarantee you'll never leave a session in a bad mood!

- ▶ Promotes relief of stress and tension through deep relaxation
- ▶ Calms the mind and helps restore mental alertness
- ▶ Revitalizes energy and enhances nerve response
- ▶ Improves circulation throughout the body

- ▶ Encourages balance and harmony of all body systems
- ▶ Helps reduce pain in the feet and the entire body
- ▶ Promotes looser, more flexible, more fully functional feet
- ▶ Can provide effective palliative care for migraines, chemotherapy treatment, menstrual pain, sciatica, and more

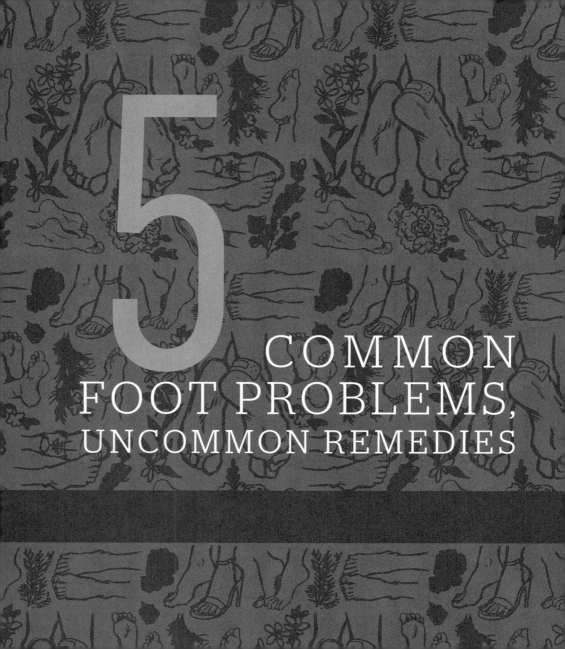

5

COMMON
FOOT PROBLEMS,
UNCOMMON REMEDIES

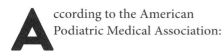

According to the American Podiatric Medical Association:

Foot ailments are among the most common of our health problems. Although some can be traced to heredity, many stem from the cumulative impact of a lifetime of abuse and neglect.

Studies show that 75 percent of Americans experience foot problems of a greater or lesser degree of seriousness at some time in their lives; nowhere near that many seek medical treatment, apparently because they mistakenly believe that discomfort and pain are normal and expectable.

Healthy feet are happy feet! Locate your foot problem(s) in the following pages and try the recommended natural remedies and basic care suggestions to help put your feet back on the path to comfort and wellness.

Arthritis

Arthritis is the inflammation of a joint, usually accompanied by pain, swelling, stiffness, and frequently changes in structure and function. Osteoarthritis, the most common form of this disease, is often the result of years of daily joint stress and accumulated injury.

Symptoms include stiffness and pain in the joints after heavy exercise, during damp or cold weather, or after long periods of inactivity. The 33 small joints in each foot and ankle are particularly vulnerable due to the load they must carry daily.

Gout, once called the "disease of kings," is a form of arthritis that tends to affect men of middle age and older who eat overly rich food, drink alcohol, and are somewhat overweight. Characteristically, gout produces sudden and severe attacks of pain and swelling triggered by excess uric acid in the blood that crystallizes in the tissues

---

FOOT NOTE
Your feet often mirror your general health, so they may be the first part of your body to exhibit symptoms for conditions like arthritis, diabetes, and nerve and circulatory disorders.

around the joints, forming an inflamed bump, usually at the base of the big toe, though other joints are susceptible.

TREATMENT Arthritis is often incurable, but the pain can be somewhat relieved with appropriate natural treatments, such as the Soothing Herbal Poultice (page 52) and Sweet Relief Arthritis Rub (page 53).

I find that consuming a strong cup of ginger tea daily helps tremendously with occasional pain from arthritis, as does taking a supplement containing black pepper, cayenne, ginger, Indian frankincense, rosemary, and turmeric—these herbs act as natural anti-inflammatories and pain relievers.

If gout is giving you grief, try adding a couple of small glasses of unsweetened tart cherry juice to your daily diet. (Sweet cherry juice is lower in antioxidants and doesn't work as well.) It's a traditional remedy for any type of arthritic pain, but it's especially effective for gout. It helps lower uric acid levels and boosts antioxidant levels, which may help lessen the number of gout attacks. Consuming fresh apple juice and lots of water are recommended, too.

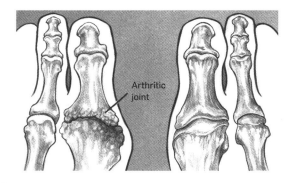

Arthritic joint

PREVENTION

▶ Wear properly fitted shoes that don't put pressure on your joints. Many sufferers benefit from full-length gel insoles.

▶ When your foot joints are particularly stiff and inflamed, try to rest and stay off your feet until they feel better.

▶ Keep an eye on your weight. Extra pounds stress the joints and can lead to foot problems.

▶ Moderate exercise (depending on the severity of your arthritis), such as walking, swimming, or bicycling, combined with yoga, tai chi, or full-body stretching exercises will help keep joints mobile and lubricated and your body limber. Joints tend to stiffen when we are sedentary, so it is important to keep as active as possible.

▸ Make a habit of having good posture. This keeps your body weight evenly distributed over each foot.

▸ Eat a healthful diet that emphasizes whole, unprocessed foods and avoids foods that can trigger inflammation, especially if you suffer from gout. Avoid excessive caffeine and alcohol, and don't use tobacco (you already knew that one!).

MEDICAL ADVICE If your feet are normally healthy but you notice joint stiffness, tenderness, or swelling and the home treatments suggested above simply aren't helping, or if your minor arthritis takes a turn for the worse and walking becomes increasingly painful and your joints become red or inflamed, make an appointment with your health-care provider.

Ginger Tea for What Ails You

I often make ginger tea when I'm feeling achy. It's easy to make, really helps with pain, and is just so dang good.

Bring 2 cups of water to a boil in a small pan. Remove from the heat. Add 2 tablespoons of finely minced fresh ginger, cover, and let steep for 20 minutes.

Pour into a mug (there's no need to strain) and add a big squeeze of lemon and raw honey to taste. The tea tastes like ginger lemonade and is excellent hot or iced. It's also wonderful for settling an upset stomach.

SOOTHING HERBAL POULTICE

This wonderful herbal remedy helps relieve pain, stiffness, and inflammation, while also revving up circulation, which can often become stagnant in swollen, arthritic joints. It works well for any arthritic joint, though we'll focus here on the feet. The poultice is easier to apply if you have someone helping. If you're treating both feet, double the recipe.

WHAT YOU NEED

2 teaspoons powdered marshmallow root

2 teaspoons dried or powdered meadowsweet flowers

2 teaspoons dried plantain leaves

½ teaspoon powdered cayenne pepper

Boiling water (about ¼ cup)

Flaxseed/rice heating bag or small electric heating pad

A doubled-over piece of cotton flannel large enough to cover your foot

Gallon-size or larger plastic bag

CONTRAINDICATION

Meadowsweet contains natural salicylic acid; do not use this recipe if you are allergic to aspirin or taking prescription blood thinners.

1 Combine the herbs in a small bowl. Add boiling water a little at a time, stirring until you have a gooey paste that feels slippery (this will happen quickly). Be careful not to add so much water that the mixture becomes runny. Allow to cool until the mixture is comfortable to touch.

2 While the mixture cools, warm the heating bag in the microwave or set the heating pad on medium heat. Soak the flannel in very warm water and wring it out.

3 Sit in a comfortable chair where you can elevate your feet. Spread the paste thickly on the affected joint. Cover the paste with the warm, damp flannel and put your foot in the plastic bag. Put the heating bag or pad on your foot and relax for at least 30 minutes (if you're using a heating bag, you will probably need to reheat it once or twice, which is another reason to have an assistant).

4 Rinse the poultice off your foot and dry well. When you're done, massage a good, thick cream (one with peppermint is especially nice) into your feet. Then put on socks.

Note: Safe for folks 6 years of age and older

SWEET RELIEF ARTHRITIS RUB

YIELD

1 treatment

WHAT YOU NEED

1–2 teaspoons castor oil or St. John's wort–infused oil

2 drops ginger essential oil

2 drops lavender essential oil

The two base oil options in this recipe both offer soothing, anti-inflammatory properties. I like castor oil's viscous texture and gently warming nature. St. John's wort–infused oil (available from many natural foods stores and herbal companies), with its gorgeous red hue, is one of my go-to herbal remedies to effectively comfort the smaller joints when they are experiencing sharp or throbbing pain. Ginger adds a circulatory-enhancing, analgesic boost for sore joints, and lavender calms and relaxes. It's great for comforting arthritic hands, too.

Mix all the ingredients thoroughly in a very small bowl. Gently massage into the areas of your feet and ankles that are affected by arthritis.

When you're finished, wipe any excess oil from your feet, or don a pair of socks and let it all soak in.

Note: Safe for folks 12 years of age and older; for children aged 6–11, use only 2 drops of essential oil

Athlete's Foot

Athlete's foot, a common fungal skin infection, is so named because it is often seen on the feet of athletes, who spend time around swimming pools, communal steam baths and showers, and locker rooms, where the infection is easily spread. Nearly 70 percent of the population deals with this infection at some point, though it is particularly prevalent among men and adolescent boys.

The dermatophytes (parasitic fungi) that cause athlete's foot thrive in warm, moist places, including closed-toe shoes and outdoor soil. Dermatophytes are opportunistic and will take advantage of any weakness that will allow them to proliferate, such as cracks in the skin or lowered immunity. They can also cause ringworm and jock itch, as well as fingernail and toenail fungal infections.

Sometimes appearing rather quickly, symptoms can include peeling or cracking of the skin between the toes and on the soles of the feet, plus intense itching, heat, redness, and dryness. If the disease is allowed to progress without treatment, it can lead to blisters, bacterial infection, and even ulcers. Athlete's foot symptoms tend to recur easily once you've been infected.

Diabetics are especially prone to athlete's foot. The abundance of glucose in their perspiration is the perfect feeding ground for fungi, allowing them to proliferate.

TREATMENT A cure for this miserable skin affliction is sometimes elusive because the pesky fungi live in the top layers of the skin and can be difficult to reach with topical treatments. Even oral prescription medications are not always effective. All treatments for athlete's foot *must* be applied or taken continuously over a period of several weeks to several months. Consistency is key to eradicating the fungus! With any treatment, forgo using nail polish until the fungus is gone.

Go herbal. Simple, effective herbal remedies do exist. If your toenails appear to have a fungal infection, apply 1 drop of tea tree essential oil to each affected toenail, twice daily. Massage in well. This treatment alone is often quite effective, and it helps clear fungus from between the toes, too.

Usnea (a lichen), black walnut hull, and oregano all have antifungal properties. They are easy to apply as tinctures (alcohol extracts, available from better natural foods stores and online purveyors of herbal products). To use, wash your feet with warm, soapy water and dry them thoroughly. Massage a dropperful (or more, if needed) of your chosen tincture into the affected areas. It should quickly soak into the skin.

Next, apply a thin coating of Happy Feet Antifungal Drops (page 59)—the tinctures alone can be too drying to the skin. Follow this procedure twice daily. I've seen this double treatment work wonders for stubborn cases of athlete's foot.

Get some garlic. Garlic is considered a potent medicinal food, effective against a broad spectrum of bacteria, viruses, and fungi, and it can be used topically and orally in the war against athlete's foot. Allicin, ajoene, and other organosulfur constituents are responsible for its remedial action and odor.

Garlic oil is readily available in capsule form. Simply pierce two to four capsules (depending on the size of the affected area) and rub the oil into your feet once or twice per day, then put on socks.

Garlic capsules can be taken orally to boost your immune system and fight the battle from the inside. Follow the manufacturer's directions for dosage, and make sure to take the capsules with food and a large glass of water. If you love cooking with garlic, feel free to add it liberally to your food. Gently sautéing it for 10 minutes releases the vital antifungal chemicals.

Garlic has a tendency to upset sensitive stomachs and cause gas, so you be the judge as to what your tolerance level is. The only issue with garlic is that you inherit the lovely fumes along with the benefits. (A neat trick for removing the odor is to rub your hands on a stainless steel sink or other stainless steel object. Works like magic!)

Try vinegar. Many of my clients have had much success with daily vinegar foot soaks. Vinegar's antifungal properties are effective against mild forms of athlete's foot and toenail fungus and help soothe dry, cracked, scaly feet.

Combine 1 part apple cider vinegar with 2 parts warm water in a foot-soaking basin. You only need enough to cover the soles of your feet and toes.

Avoid Contagion

Athlete's foot can be spread by contact with an infected person or from contact with contaminated surfaces, such as towels, floors, and bathmats. If you are dealing with athlete's foot, avoid spreading the fungus by drying your feet with paper towels or with hand towels that you use once and then launder in hot water.

Do not use a bathmat if you share a bathroom with other people. Use a clean towel every time you bathe and wash towels in hot water between uses. Clean your shower/tub floor regularly with a 10 percent bleach solution or a commercial disinfectant to kill any resident fungi.

Soak your feet for 20 minutes. Yes, the odor is strong, but it dissipates as your feet dry. Follow with an application of Happy Feet Antifungal Drops (page 59).

PREVENTION

- Wash your feet twice daily in warm, soapy water. Dry thoroughly.
- Change your socks, hosiery, and shoes during the day if you perspire heavily.
- Wear open-toe shoes as often as possible. Your feet can breathe and stay drier this way.
- Expose your feet to warm sunshine and fresh air as much as possible.
- Allow your shoes to air out and dry between wearings to minimize fungal proliferation.
- Apply antifungal powder to your feet each day to keep sweat at bay and prevent the fungus from spreading.

- Wear shower shoes or rubber thongs when using public showers, walking in locker rooms and around public swimming pools, or lounging in a steam room.
- Clean all nail-trimming implements with disinfectant and don't share them with friends or other family members.
- If you have professional pedicures, choose a nail salon that uses sterilized manicure tools for each customer, or better yet, bring your own.
- Limit your consumption of refined carbohydrates and high-glycemic foods such as white sugar, white rice, white flour, white potatoes, chips, pretzels, dried fruit, honey, and supersweet fresh fruits. This is not only good dietary advice in general, it also keeps fungal growth at bay.
- Keep an eye on your weight, which can exacerbate perspiration. People who sweat a lot are more prone to athlete's foot.

MEDICAL ADVICE If self-treatment is not helping after a few weeks, make an appointment with your healthcare provider or podiatrist to rule out other skin problems that can masquerade as athlete's foot, such as dermatitis or problems resulting from diabetes, circulatory disorders, drug abuse, medicine side effects, or a vitamin or mineral deficiency. If necessary, your healthcare provider can prescribe topical or oral antifungal medications to use in conjunction with the above treatments and preventive measures. As with any medication, please ask questions about potential side effects; antifungal drugs can be toxic to the liver.

YIELD

2 cups

WHAT YOU NEED

1 cup baking soda

½ cup cornstarch or arrowroot powder

½ cup white cosmetic clay (also known as powdered white clay or kaolin)

100 drops eucalyptus, geranium, lavender, tea tree, and/or thyme essential oil (I like a 50:50 combination of geranium and lavender)

Shaker containers (glass, plastic, or cardboard)

FUNGUS FIGHTER FOOT POWDER

I make my own foot and body powders because they're so simple to create and the ingredients can be customized to suit my needs and fragrance preferences. This powder smells clean, keeps odor and moisture at bay, and is recommended as part of your daily arsenal in the fight against foot fungus.

1 Combine the baking soda, cornstarch, and white clay in a medium bowl and gently mix with a whisk. Add the essential oil(s) a few drops at a time, whisking as you go. (You can also pulse the dry ingredients in a food processor and continue pulsing as you add the essential oil.)

2 Transfer the powder to an airtight container and store in a dark, cool place for 3 days to allow the essential oil's fragrance and remedial properties to permeate the mixture.

3 Package the blend in small shaker containers. Label and date. Store at room temperature, away from heat and light; use within 1 year.

To use, sprinkle the powder into your socks once or twice daily, or apply to dry, bare feet.

Note: Safe for folks 6 years of age and older; if pregnant or breastfeeding, avoid eucalyptus and thyme essential oils

YIELD

2 ounces

WHAT YOU NEED

15 drops geranium essential oil

13 drops lavender essential oil

10 drops tea tree essential oil

5 drops lemon essential oil

5 drops thyme essential oil

2-ounce dark glass bottle with a dropper top

¼ cup almond, extra-virgin olive, fractionated coconut, jojoba, or castor oil

HAPPY FEET ANTIFUNGAL DROPS

This herbal oil blend, with its rather pleasing medicinal aroma, works double duty. In addition to helping to eradicate the scourge of athlete's foot and nail fungus, it also calms and soothes redness and itching, conditions cracked or peeling skin, and fights odor.

Combine the essential oils in the glass bottle, then add your base oil of choice. Screw the top on the bottle and shake vigorously for 2 minutes to blend. Label and date the bottle, and set it in a cool, dark location for 24 hours so that the oils can synergize. Store at room temperature, away from heat and light; use within 1 year (2 years if you used jojoba oil as your base).

To use, shake the bottle well and apply a few drops to clean, dry feet. Apply to both feet, even if only one is affected. Massage in thoroughly, being sure to get oil between the toes and on the toenails. Allow the oil to penetrate for a few minutes and then put on socks. Repeat the application twice daily for several months, or until the condition abates.

Caution: This is a concentrated formula, so use it only by the drop, as directed, and wash your hands after applying.

Note: Safe for folks 12 years of age and older; for children aged 6–11, reduce the essential oils by half; if pregnant or breastfeeding, replace thyme essential oil with additional tea tree essential oil

Black Toenail

A black toenail, or subungual hematoma, stems from an injury that causes blood to pool under the nail. The bruise can vary from a small dot to covering the entire toenail. The accumulated blood may eventually press on nerves, often resulting in pain, at least temporarily. With a severe or repeated injury, the toenail may loosen or even detach.

Possible causes include trauma, such as stubbing the toe or dropping something heavy on it, or accumulated stress from wearing shoes that are much too short or activities, such as hiking, tennis, or soccer, in which the toes repeatedly jam up against the end of the shoe. Runners experience this malady so frequently that it is sometimes referred to as runner's toenail.

TREATMENT In the case of an acute injury, the toenail can usually be saved if the blood is drained within 48 hours following injury. This procedure might make you a bit woozy (I get dizzy just thinking about it!), but if you're brave and have a steady hand, it is worth attempting.

First, clean your foot thoroughly, dry it off, and swab the affected toe with at least 70 percent rubbing alcohol.

Next, heat the end of a needle, a very fine drill bit, or the tip of an unbent paperclip with a match until it is red hot. Immediately, but gently, pierce your toenail just until blood is released.

The heat from the sharp object melts the hard keratin protein of the nail and allows the blood to flow out from beneath. There are no nerves in the nail itself, so you will feel no pain unless you pierce through to the nail bed.

Follow this procedure with a warm footbath to which you've added ½ cup of either table salt or sea salt. Soak for 15 minutes. Dry your feet and swab the toe with 70 percent rubbing alcohol or a disinfectant herbal tincture, such as usnea, oregano, or echinacea, and then apply a drop of tea tree essential oil.

If your toenail *does* begin to loosen over time, cushion the nail with gauze and tape it down with an adhesive bandage (don't stick tape directly to the nail itself or you may rip the nail off when you remove the bandage). This prevents your toenail from catching on your hosiery or socks.

Caution: Never perform this type of self-treatment if you have circulatory disorders or are diabetic. Instead, see your healthcare provider or podiatrist immediately.

If you suffer from chronically bruised and blackened toenails, you can leave them alone if they don't bother you. If they do, soaking in a warm footbath to which you've added ½ cup of Epsom salts or sea salt may relieve some of the discomfort.

PREVENTION Other than trying to be more graceful and not drop things on your toes, be sure to buy properly fitting shoes, especially for athletic endeavors.

MEDICAL ADVICE If you can't bring yourself to puncture your own nail, a visit to your healthcare provider or podiatrist to perform the procedure will save you downtime and avoid complications such as excessive swelling and possible infection.

Blisters

Everyone has experienced a blister at one time or another. They are caused by excessive friction and pressure on the skin and can develop on any part of the foot, including the tips of the toes, especially if the foot is swollen. Any type of footwear can cause a blister, though shoes that are too short or too narrow are more likely to do so. Active folks tend to suffer more blisters than sedentary folks, particularly distance runners/walkers and those who have jobs that require a lot of walking.

You can actually feel a blister beginning to form. The spot becomes warm, then irritated, then downright painful if you don't remove your shoe. A whitish pocket of skin filled with clear fluid forms just beneath the top layer of skin in response to the irritation and can make walking unbearable. When the fluid is mixed with blood, it is called a blood blister and will appear quite dark.

TREATMENT There are different schools of thought on whether or not to pop a blister. Many healthcare providers say to leave it alone, especially if it is small to medium in size and the pain is minimal. After eliminating the source of friction, wash the area and swab it with 70 percent rubbing alcohol or another disinfectant. Ice it for 15 minutes or so to help minimize pain and swelling, then pat the area dry and cover it with an adhesive bandage or moleskin. Most blisters will drain on their own within a few days.

Other medical professionals and sports injury specialists suggest that popping a blister, particularly a larger, more painful one, will allow it to heal more quickly. (And if a blister breaks on its own, you would treat it the same as if you had popped it intentionally.)

To pop or open a blister, wash the area and swab it with 70 percent rubbing alcohol or another disinfectant. Carefully puncture the edge of the blister with a sterilized needle (use a flame or alcohol to sterilize it or boil it for at least 5 minutes) or sterile lancet or razor blade.

Drain the fluid using gentle pressure, but don't peel off any skin. Allow the layers of skin to adhere. Cleanse the area with disinfectant again and pat dry.

Apply commercial antibiotic ointment or two drops of castor oil mixed with a drop or two of tea tree essential oil. Apply a bandage. Remove the bandage at night to allow the blister to breathe and dry out and put on a new one in the morning (and after you shower or bathe). A new layer of skin will form under the blister, and eventually the skin from the original blister will fall away.

Caution: Don't attempt to pop a large blister if you have circulatory problems or are diabetic; instead see your healthcare provider, podiatrist, or certified foot care nurse immediately.

PREVENTION

- Purchase well-fitting shoes that do not rub anywhere, right from the initial wearing. Add soft insoles or heel cushions made from foam or gel, if necessary.
- If you are prone to blisters or physically active, always wear good socks and apply adhesive felt or moleskin to susceptible areas on your feet.
- To reduce friction, sprinkle powder into your socks or rub it into your bare feet daily. Fungus Fighter Foot Powder (page 58) and Odor-Neutralizing Herbal Foot Powder (page 111) are great everyday foot powders.

- Some active folks swear by petroleum jelly, plain vegetable shortening, diaper rash balm with zinc oxide, calendula salve, tincture of benzoin, or even old-fashioned Vicks VapoRub as effective topical lubricants to prevent blisters. Medical-grade hydrogel pads (2nd Skin is a good brand) work great, too. Quickie Blister Resister Oil Blend (page 64) is my go-to formula that I've used for many years.

MEDICAL ADVICE Blisters are rarely serious, but an infected one can cause more serious complications, such as cellulitis. Please see your healthcare provider or podiatrist immediately if a blister isn't healing after a few days.

YIELD

4 ounces

WHAT YOU NEED

12 drops lavender
essential oil

6 drops copaiba
essential oil

6 drops tea tree
essential oil

4-ounce bottle
castor oil

QUICKIE BLISTER RESISTER OIL BLEND

With viscous castor oil as the base, this blend effectively lubricates, conditions, and soothes the skin, minimizing potential friction and inflammation.

Add the essential oils directly to the castor oil bottle. Screw the top on the bottle and shake vigorously for 2 minutes to blend. Label and date the bottle and set it in a cool, dark location for 24 hours so that the oils can synergize. Store in a cool, dark cabinet, and use within 1 year.

Shake the bottle well before each use. Apply the oil to blister-prone areas, then put on socks.

Note: Safe for folks 6 years of age and older; for children aged 2–5, reduce the essential oils by half

Bunions

Humans are not born with bunions. Although they seem to run in families, there's no "bunion gene." Foot shape and structure *are* hereditary, however, and some foot types are more prone to bunions than others. People with low arches, flat feet, loose joints and tendons, limb length discrepancy, hip misalignment, overpronation, foot deformities, and arthritic joint destruction are all at increased risk, as are overweight individuals.

Fitting young children in shoes that are widest at the balls of the feet as opposed to where they are naturally widest, at the toes, is when the potential for bunion deformity truly begins.

A bunion, or hallux valgus, is a dislocation of the first metatarsal head (the joint at the base of the big toe). Inflammation and thickening of the small fluid-filled bursa in this area are accompanied by enlargement and stiffness of the joint, deformity of the toe, widening of the forefoot, and weakening and sagging of the arch.

The result is a misshapen foot, with the big toe angling in or shifting out of position toward the other toes and sometimes tucking under or over the second toe.

Bunions can become quite painful if allowed to progress. Though not as common, a similar protruding bump at the outer base of the fifth (little) toe, called a bunionette or tailor's bunion, can also form, with the little toe angled inward toward the big toe.

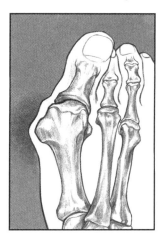

TREATMENT Switching from shoes with a pointed or even tapered toe box to shoes with a wide forefoot or open-toe sandals can help tremendously. So-called "bunion shoes," available from most orthopedic shoe stores, are designed to be soft, relatively flexible, supportive, and wide enough to take the pressure off your sore bunion. Shoes with heels are an absolute no-no, as they will aggravate an already stressed joint.

To make running and walking shoes more comfortable, you can make a slit in the shoe in the bunion area to allow for extra room and less pressure. If you overpronate—that's when the arches of the feet roll inward (medially) and downward when you're standing or walking—a commercial arch support can help temporarily take some of the weight off the bunion until it is remedied.

If the bunion is swollen and inflamed, elevate your foot and chill it for 10 to 20 minutes with an ice pack or frozen bag of corn or peas wrapped in a thin towel to protect your skin from direct contact. Remove the ice for 15 minutes, then repeat.

If the bunion really aches at the end of the day, you can treat your feet while you sleep by wearing an orthopedic bunion corrector sock or sleeve that aims to gently restore alignment of the first metatarsal, thus relieving pain. Regularly wearing toe separators such as YogaToes or Correct Toes can help improve the splay of your toes and aid in relieving bunion pain.

Topical application of a quality CBD oil works wonders for many folks. A few drops massaged into the bunion and surrounding area twice per day can often deliver effective pain relief.

Foot exercises can also help. Perform as many of the exercises in Chapter 2 as you can daily, to the best of your ability.

Schedule weekly foot reflexology sessions, if possible. Because bunions contribute to tension and pain in the rest of the foot and lower leg, these treatments will help loosen tight, stiff feet, improve flexibility in the feet and ankles, and soothe any lower leg discomfort. A session with a massage therapist can also help release tension and provide comfort.

PREVENTION

- If bunions run in your family or you suspect the beginning stages of a bunion, you can dramatically slow the progression by wearing properly fitted shoes to prevent further misalignment.
- Avoid wearing flip-flops or any backless shoes, which cause your toes to grip and pinch in order to keep the shoes from falling off. This constant action will encourage and/or worsen a bunion.
- Last, but perhaps most important, go barefoot in grass or on soft surfaces as often as you can to keep your feet strong and flexible.

MEDICAL ADVICE If home treatments don't provide relief, a chiropractor, osteopath, or physical therapist who specializes in extremity realignment or sports rehabilitation may be able to help relieve moderate bunion pain. If you feel you need additional medical help, a visit to a podiatrist is in order. They may prescribe orthotics or shoe inserts to give support to the rest of the foot, though these measures will not fix the bunion. Surgery may be necessary in extreme cases. Your doctor may want to rule out osteoarthritis, rheumatoid arthritis, or gout, as these can also cause pain and inflammation in the big toe.

Calluses

A common malady, calluses are simply a buildup or accumulation of skin cells or keratinocytes in the outermost layer of skin, primarily over bony prominences of the foot. They're thick, tough, and hard, develop in various shapes and sizes, and can form anywhere on the bottom of your foot, your heel, the medial side of your big toe, or even the tops and tips of your toes as a defense mechanism against repeated friction and pressure. They can become painful if allowed to grow very thick.

Anything that causes excessive friction, pressure, or pinching of the skin on your foot can result in a callus, including shoes that are too tight, too short, or even too big and floppy. Going barefoot a lot often leads to callus formation. Additionally, a gait imbalance due to injury, limping, or structural misalignment can promote callusing on the feet because normal, balanced walking is compromised. Most people develop them at some point in their life.

TREATMENT The only way to permanently remove a callus is to remove the cause. Calluses return, no matter how often you scrape and file them off. They keep pedicurists in business.

As an advocate of barefoot life, I tend to my minor calluses twice a week, usually after showering or soaking in the tub. You can also soak your feet for 15 minutes in a tub of warm water to which you can add either ½ cup of raw apple cider vinegar or ½ cup of baking soda. (Don't mix them or you'll create a fizzy mess!)

After soaking, smooth the rough surfaces of any calluses with one of the following tools:

- ► Foot file with medium-grit sandpaper on one side and fine grit on the other
- ► Plastic-handled pediwand containing an embedded pumice stone
- ► Large diamond-dust nail file
- ► Pumice stone

After smoothing your feet, dry them thoroughly and apply a thick

---

FOOT NOTE

The two most common foot problems seen by nail technicians are calluses and dry, cracked heels. These ailments appear on feet of all ages, but especially in seniors.

moisturizer or a foot balm, such as my Creamy Cocoa Butter Foot Balm (page 39), and put on socks to help the moisturizer sink in.

For particularly large or thick calluses, you can purchase a corn and callus trimmer or shaver (also known as a rasp) that uses a small razor blade to scrape off layers of softened callus. Use this tool with extreme caution so that you do not cut too deeply and draw blood. A safer alternative is a small battery-operated callus remover that gently grinds calluses and collects the debris in a cup for disposal.

Commercial foot scrubs made with sugar or salt are also popular and effective if you have minor callusing. Or try one of my easy-to-make home versions: Sweet Feet Sugary Foot Scrub (page 70) and Peppermint Salt Glo (page 71).

For people with especially tough feet, commercial exfoliating foot creams that contain ingredients such as lactates (ammonium, sodium, or potassium), lactic acid, salicylic acid, glycolic acid, urea, hyaluronic acid, ceramides, shea butter, and glycerin will help keep feet nice and smooth. Follow the directions for use on the package.

Caution: Diabetics, people with circulatory problems, and those with unsteady hands should never attempt to cut or scrape their calluses with tools containing blades.

PREVENTION

▸ Take good care of your feet. Inspect them frequently for developing calluses and other foot problems and treat accordingly.
▸ Wear quality shoes and socks that fit. No rubbing or binding allowed.
▸ If you're overweight, please work on paring the pounds. Excess weight puts way too much pressure on the small joints in your feet and encourages callus formation.

MEDICAL ADVICE If your calluses are not responding to home treatment and become painful, see a podiatrist, certified foot care nurse, or master pedicurist. Calluses can form because of a foot/ankle misalignment (or a misalignment elsewhere in the body), which would need to be treated. In this case, you might seek out a chiropractor, osteopath, or physical therapist who specializes in extremity realignment or sports rehabilitation.

YIELD

1 treatment

WHAT YOU NEED

¼ cup granulated white or brown sugar

2 tablespoons almond, extra-virgin olive, fractionated coconut, or jojoba oil

6 drops ginger, grape-fruit, spearmint, and/or sweet orange essential oil

SWEET FEET SUGARY FOOT SCRUB

This simple, aromatic sugar scrub yields supersoft feet.

1 Combine all the ingredients in a small bowl and mix thoroughly.

2 Soak and wash your feet to soften the callused skin. Pat dry. While sitting on the edge of the tub or over a towel or foot-soaking basin, massage half of the sugar mixture into one foot, scrubbing with a moderately firm hand over your callused areas for at least 2 to 3 minutes. Repeat on your other foot.

3 Rinse with warm water and roughly rub your feet dry. There should be a little bit of oily residue remaining on your feet that will penetrate and continue to soften your skin for hours to come.

If you really want to pamper your feet, after the scrub, massage a bit of your favorite foot cream or a bit of castor oil into each foot and then put on a pair of socks.

Note: Safe for folks over 2 years of age

PEPPERMINT SALT GLO

This invigorating, cooling, refreshing scrub is sure to awaken and enliven your senses!

YIELD

1 treatment

WHAT YOU NEED

¼ cup sea salt or table salt

2 tablespoons almond, extra-virgin olive, fractionated coconut, or jojoba oil

6 drops peppermint essential oil

1 Combine all the ingredients in a small bowl and mix thoroughly.

2 Soak and wash your feet to soften the callused skin. Pat dry. While sitting on the edge of the tub or over a towel or foot-soaking basin, massage half of the salt mixture into one foot, scrubbing with a moderately firm hand over your callused areas for at least 2 to 3 minutes. Repeat on your other foot.

3 Rinse with warm water and roughly rub your feet dry. There should be a little bit of oily residue remaining on your feet that will penetrate and continue to soften your skin for hours to come.

   If you really want to pamper your feet, after the scrub, massage a bit of your favorite foot cream or a bit of castor oil into each foot and then put on a pair of socks.

Note: Safe for folks over 2 years of age; if pregnant or breastfeeding, replace peppermint essential oil with lavender, lemon, or grapefruit essential oil

Cold Feet

There are a variety of causes for cold feet, and women tend to suffer from them more than men. Is it because many women often wear tight, fashionable shoes that restrict circulation to the feet? That's certainly one reason.

Cold feet can also be the result of side effects from certain medications, high blood pressure, iron deficiency anemia, cardiovascular disease, liver disease, kidney disease, diabetes, Raynaud's disease, hypothyroidism, nerve disorders, low muscle mass, trauma, injury, smoking, high stress, anxiety, or a sedentary lifestyle. And, obviously, being out in low temperatures in poorly insulated shoes will leave you with cold feet.

Whatever the cause, cold feet can be downright annoying, uncomfortable, and sometimes painful. They are sometimes tingly and a bit numb, and they can even be a bit bluish or purple in color due to poor circulation. A chronic case can lead to dry skin that is prone to cracking and deeper fissures.

TREATMENT Walk, walk, walk! Keep those feet moving and your heart pumping. The more you move, the better your circulation, which is the key to warm feet. Don't like walking or are unable to do so? Then purchase a rebounder (mini-trampoline) for your home, try yoga or Pilates, swim at the gym, or follow an online or prerecorded exercise class. Just *move*!

One of the quickest ways to relieve cold feet is to soak them for 15 to 20 minutes in a warm footbath. I like to add ½ cup of Epsom salts to help relax foot muscles. This is especially wonderful just before bed because it drains tension from the body and prepares the nervous system for sleep. Placing your feet on a heating pad, hot water bottle, or microwavable flax/rice heating bag is also comforting.

Wearing warm socks is important for folks with cold feet. Indoors, wear well-insulated slippers, especially if you don't have carpeted or heated floors. Cold feet can drain the heat from the rest of the body . . . brrr!

Dietary changes might help. For example, eat foods containing vitamins A, B complex, C, D, and E, as well as bioflavonoids and iron (unless contraindicated by your healthcare provider). These nutrients strengthen the veins and capillaries and help keep your blood oxygen rich. Spicy substances—hot sauce, chiles, ginger, cinnamon, cloves, oregano, thyme, and rosemary—can rev up your circulation as well.

Think about scheduling some reflexology or massage sessions to improve circulation and reduce tension in your feet and legs.

PREVENTION

▸ Always wear comfortable shoes, never ones that are too tight or too short.
▸ Keep your feet warm and dry by wearing socks that breathe; natural fibers or quality synthetic will do, as long as they wick excess moisture away from your feet.
▸ Maintain an active lifestyle as best you can.
▸ Eat a nutritious, well-balanced, whole-foods diet and drink plenty of water.
▸ If you sit or stand in one position all day long, be sure to stretch your feet and legs periodically to keep blood from stagnating in your legs.

MEDICAL ADVICE Getting cold feet from time to time is perfectly normal, but persistent symptoms are another matter. If none of the above suggestions seem to help, schedule a visit to your healthcare provider or a podiatrist to rule out anything serious.

Heating Herbal Powders

You may have heard this oldie-but-goodie remedy: Sprinkle powdered cayenne or ginger into your socks for a warming effect. Both are considered stimulating, heating herbs that promote increased circulation when in contact with the skin. But I wouldn't recommend them undiluted.

Instead, mix ½ to 1 teaspoon of either herb with about 2 teaspoons of white cosmetic clay, cornstarch, or arrowroot, and then sprinkle away. Be sure to wash your hands thoroughly after handling the mixture. Note that the cayenne will stain light-colored socks and may sting any open cuts, scrapes, or insect bites.

YIELD

1 treatment

WHAT YOU NEED

1–2 teaspoons almond, extra-virgin olive, fractionated coconut, jojoba, or castor oil

4 drops black pepper, clove, frankincense, ginger, rosemary, and/ or thyme essential oil

WARM-ME-UP FOOT RUB

This easy-to-make blend contains essential oils valued for their heating and circulation-stimulating properties. Perfect therapy for cold feet!

Mix all the ingredients thoroughly in a very small bowl. Gently massage into your feet and ankles for a few minutes. This will make your hands nice and warm, too! Be careful not to rub any into your eyes or nose, as this blend may irritate mucous membranes.

When you're finished, wipe any excess oil from your feet, or don a pair of socks and let it all soak in.

Note: Safe for folks 12 years of age and older; for children aged 6–11, use only 2 drops of essential oil; if pregnant or breastfeeding, avoid clove, rosemary, and thyme essential oils

Corns

Corns are hard, thick, round, generally smooth, and pale yellowish to fleshy colored. They are about the size of a kernel of corn or smaller. They are caused by pressure or friction on the tips or tops of the toes or even, if your toes are rubbing together, between them. Corns can also occur on the bottom of the feet, where they can be confused with plantar warts.

People with extremely high arches are often susceptible because their toes are contracted downward, giving them a "clawing deformity" such as you see with hammertoe or claw toe conditions; their toes bend at the center, increasing the potential for friction against the tops of their shoes.

Unlike a wart, a corn does not contain capillaries or nerve endings, but it can press on underlying nerve endings,

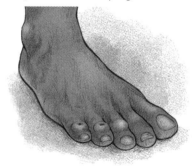

often causing discomfort or even sharp, stabbing pain while you are walking.

A hard corn (heloma durum) is a thickening of the horny (outer) layer of the epidermis, exhibiting a tough, inverted cone shape with a brownish gray "eye" or central core, surrounded by inflammation. A soft corn (heloma molle) forms between the toes, where dampness softens the normally hard corn tissue. The constant friction between your toes can cause the skin of a soft corn to become inflamed.

TREATMENT You can either start wearing better-fitting shoes that don't squeeze your feet, taking the pressure off your corns so they'll go away on their own, or you can perform constant maintenance on your existing and new corns.

Corn pads have a hole cut out of the middle so the padding fits around the corn and relieves any pressure on it. Corn pads take up space, so make sure to wear roomier shoes while wearing the pad. Medicated corn disks, impregnated with salicylic acid, encourage the corn to peel and shed its tough layers.

Custom pads can also be made from moleskin or adhesive felt, as thick as you wish, but always put the padding around the corn, not on top of it.

Salicylic ointment or drops (also known as corn drops) can be applied directly to a corn to help peel it away, but if any of the acid runs off onto the surrounding skin, with repeated application, it can burn and even cause a hole or ulcer to form. The drops can be applied in the center of a corn pad, but please use them with care.

Caution: Diabetics should never use salicylic acid products to treat a corn. Ulceration of the skin could lead to serious problems.

Other remedies that work for some folks include applying raw apple cider vinegar to the corn twice daily. The acetic acid softens tough skin and encourages peeling. Castor oil can also be applied to help soften the skin and reduce inflammation. After dabbing either of these on the corn, cover it with a bandage. Repeat twice daily for 30 days. Consistency is the key to

success, but if you see no improvement after this period, try another treatment.

You can also try placing lambswool, either natural or synthetic, between your toes as padding while a corn heals.

PREVENTION

- ▶ Stop wearing shoes that pinch, bind, compress, or are too short.
- ▶ Wear open-toe sandals or comfortable shoes with a wide toe box.
- ▶ Go barefoot as often as possible on a comfortable surface so your feet can expand and relax.

MEDICAL ADVICE If a corn reaches the painful stage and nothing seems to be helping, a podiatrist, master pedicurist, or certified foot care nurse may use a blade to carefully shave away the thickened, dead skin, or they may choose to apply a potent exfoliating product. Be aware that the corn is almost certain to return if you continue to wear the same shoe styles.

Diabetic Foot Concerns

Diabetics often suffer from foot problems such as neuropathy, numbness, tingling, burning, swelling, foot odor, dry skin, fissures, ulceration, calluses, and corns. Like everyone else, diabetics can also have a problem with athlete's foot and toenail fungus—the increased glucose in their blood creates "sweet" perspiration that encourages fungal infection.

Sensory diabetic neuropathy is the gradual loss of nerve function in the legs and feet, leading to a loss of feeling or sensation and impaired functioning of the muscles. It can also affect the ankles and hands. If you have this disease, you won't be able to feel if you've injured your foot or if blisters have formed from snug shoes. Loss of feeling in the feet can lead to serious problems.

Peripheral vascular disease or poor circulation in the limbs can slow the healing process. What might start as a minor cut, bruise, blister, corn, or callus could develop into an open sore, infection, ulceration, and eventually gangrene if not properly cared for.

Diabetics frequently suffer from cold feet and hands, too.

See the specific ailments described in this chapter for treatment suggestions, but it is wise for diabetics to visit a podiatrist or certified foot care nurse at least every 3 months to prevent any minor problems from developing into potentially limb-threatening complications.

TREATMENT Treating diabetic foot ailments is usually best left in the hands of a podiatrist or certified foot care nurse—too many things could go awry if home treatment is attempted. Foot care specialists do, however, recommend using a good moisturizer on the feet daily to help keep corns and calluses smooth and soft, thus heading off any potential infection caused by dry skin cracks and deeper fissures.

You can use your favorite body lotion, cream, or butter and add a couple drops of lavender, peppermint, or copaiba essential oil, if you wish. Or try your hand at whipping up a batch of Creamy Cocoa Butter Foot Balm (page 39).

Dry Skin and Poor Circulation?

These are common complaints for diabetics. A daily session of dry brushing will quickly banish scaly skin problems and improve blood and lymph flow in the legs. Using a loofah sponge and/or natural fiber body brush with a handle, start at the soles and work up to your thighs, spending 2 to 3 minutes on each leg. Follow each session by slathering on your favorite soothing moisturizer. (Be sure to wash and dry the brush at least once a week.)

PREVENTION

- ► Inspect your feet daily for developing corns, calluses, blisters, or anything unusual, such as color change, swelling, or sores that are slow to heal. Treat minor blisters, corns, and calluses immediately.

- ► Check shoes for fit and wear patterns and replace them as necessary. They should never be too tight, too narrow, or too short, since this could further impair circulation. Wear seamless socks to avoid irritation. High heels and open-toe sandals are not recommended.

- ► Wash your feet daily with mild soap and warm water, and make sure to completely dry between your toes. A blow dryer on the lowest setting does a super job of drying your feet and can be especially handy if your feet are so tender that rubbing them with a towel would cause discomfort. Afterward, dust your feet with powder to keep perspiration in check.

- Do daily foot exercises to improve circulation (see Chapter 2).
- Don't cross your legs for long periods of time.
- Don't go barefoot unless you are on carpeting or an area you know to be clear from potential hazards. (Always check with your doctor first to be sure that going barefoot is safe for you.)
- Apply moisturizer to your feet daily to keep your skin hydrated.
- If you smoke, quit! I don't need to tell you that it contributes to poor circulation and poor health in general.
- Eat a well-balanced, low-sugar, whole-foods diet, including plenty of water.
- Finally, make exercise a daily habit. Good circulation is key to keeping leg and foot complications at bay.

MEDICAL ADVICE Diabetes is a serious disease, and for diabetics, even an ordinary foot problem should not be ignored; it could be life-threatening if not dealt with promptly. Never attempt home treatments that could cause an open wound, such as cutting calluses or corns and popping blisters. Even using a pumice stone too aggressively could open the gate for infection.

Your best and safest bet for any foot problem is to visit a foot specialist, such as a podiatrist, certified foot care nurse, or your regular healthcare provider. A master pedicurist can be seen for routine foot and toenail maintenance (and a colorful slick of polish, if you desire!).

> *How beautiful are the feet of those who bring good news!*
>
> —Romans 10:15

Dry, Cracked Feet

Dry skin can affect any part of the body, but the soles of your feet are particularly susceptible because they, like the palms of your hands, lack oil glands to keep them lubricated. These glands secrete sebum, which helps prevent the evaporation of moisture from the skin.

Dry feet can result from nutritional deficiency (specifically vitamins A, B complex, C, D, E, and K), inadequate hydration, a dry environment, swimming in chlorinated pools, spending a lot of time walking barefoot, or just simple neglect. Rubbing lotion on your feet may help a bit, but basic foot care must become a daily habit.

Dry, cracked, rough, scaly skin on the feet is a common problem, especially in winter. It's not only uncomfortable and unsightly but can predispose you to infection, especially if you suffer from poor blood flow to your limbs. The entire foot can be affected, but usually the ball, heel, toe webbing, and lateral edge suffer most.

If the condition is allowed to progress, the skin tissue tends to thicken, harden, and become itchy. Small cracks may form and later develop into fissures that bleed. Walking becomes painful.

Ragged skin also snags on hosiery and bedsheets. Not a good feeling!

TREATMENT Morning and evening, apply thick cream, lotion, body butter, a slathering of castor oil, or my Cracked Skin Rescue Balm (page 83). Especially do this after bathing, when your feet are somewhat hydrated.

Twice a week, soak your feet for 10 to 15 minutes in a batch of Mineral-Rich Oatmeal Soak (page 82) or in a tub of warm water to which you've added ½ cup of raw apple cider vinegar, Epsom salts, or sea salt. Be aware that sea salt and vinegar will sting raw, cracked skin.

When your skin has softened somewhat, proceed with an exfoliation method of your choice—pediwand, foot file, pumice stone, sugar/salt scrub—to pare down and smooth your tootsies. (I recommend Sweet Feet Sugary Foot Scrub, page 70, and Peppermint Salt Glo, page 71.)

For those with especially tough, dry, cracked feet, the "big guns" in the foot product world might be warranted. Look for specialty foot creams containing a combination of ingredients such as lactates (ammonium, sodium, potassium), lactic acid, salicylic acid, glycolic acid, urea, hyaluronic acid, ceramides, shea butter, and glycerin. These creams work by loosening the bonds between hardened dead skin cells, allowing them to gently slough away, plus they intensely hydrate and condition skin tissue. Follow the directions for use on the package.

PREVENTION Don't wait until your feet reach the dreaded, terribly painful, skin-splitting stage. Regular preventive maintenance is key!

MEDICAL ADVICE If the skin on your feet has become so hard, dry, and thick that it is resistant to home treatment, a master pedicurist or certified foot care nurse can file or pare down the buildup so you can proceed with proper maintenance. Senior folks, in particular, often suffer from dry skin problems, mainly due to the inability to simply bend over and reach their feet to take care of them. Again, routine preventive maintenance is necessary.

If your feet have developed deep fissures, become inflamed, or bleed, see your podiatrist, certified foot care nurse, or healthcare provider to prevent infection from setting in. This is especially vital if you are diabetic.

FOOT NOTE
The skin on the sole of your foot is the thickest on the body. The protective plantar fat pads located on the heel and ball of the foot thin as you age. Certain diseases, such as rheumatoid arthritis and diabetes, also cause this padding to atrophy, as does putting a lot of mileage on your feet over a lifetime.

YIELD

1 treatment

WHAT YOU NEED

Foot-soaking basin filled with water (at whatever temperature you like)

2 bath towels

½ cup colloidal oatmeal or oat flour

¼ cup white cosmetic clay (also known as powdered white clay or kaolin)

Foot file, pediwand, or pumice stone

MINERAL-RICH OATMEAL SOAK

This treatment, performed every other day or so, will slowly and safely remove most of the dry, hard skin on your feet. You can then cut back to just once or twice per week as maintenance. The footbath feels particularly moisturizing and softening because of the soothing "oat milk" that's produced when finely ground oatmeal is infused in water. It's quite therapeutic for dry, crusty, cracked, itchy skin.

1 Place the basin on a towel in front of a comfortable chair. Add the oatmeal and clay and gently stir until they are dissolved. Soak your feet for at least 10 to 15 minutes, or until any tough skin has softened, but not until your feet resemble prunes.

2 Pat your feet damp-dry, then very gently use the foot file, pediwand, or pumice stone to scrub any area that is affected by calluses, corns, and dry skin, just until the top layer of tough dead skin has been removed. Rinse, then roughly dry your feet.

3 Apply a thick cream, lotion, body butter, balm, or specialty foot exfoliating cream and put on socks to help it soak in.

Caution: Diabetics should not soak their feet. Most suffer from circulatory disorders and cannot feel if the water temperature is too hot or cold. Additionally, if the skin on a diabetic's feet gets too soft, it can lead to pre-ulcerations, especially between the toes. Seek professional help, please.

Note: Safe for all ages

CRACKED SKIN RESCUE BALM

YIELD

4 ounces

WHAT YOU NEED

4 tablespoons castor oil

2 tablespoons cocoa butter

2 tablespoons refined shea butter*

10 drops myrrh essential oil

4-ounce dark glass or plastic jar

*You could use unrefined shea butter in this recipe, but its stronger fragrance will greatly reduce the already subtle aroma of the essential oil, though not its properties.

Looking for a cracked skin remedy with an incredibly creamy texture that melts at body temperature and penetrates amazingly well? This is the one for you. It has all the conditioning benefits of lanolin, without the odd smell, stickiness, and potential irritation, plus it's vegan! It has mild antiseptic, anti-inflammatory, and skin-regenerating properties. This recipe is reprinted from my best-selling book Stephanie Tourles's Essential Oils: A Beginner's Guide.

1 Combine the castor oil, cocoa butter, and shea butter in a small saucepan or double boiler over low heat and warm them until the solids are just melted. Remove from the heat and allow to cool for 5 to 10 minutes, stirring a few times to blend the mixture thoroughly.

2 Add the myrrh essential oil directly to the jar, then slowly pour in the oil mixture. Gently stir to blend. Cap, label, and date.

3 Set aside until the balm has thickened, which may take up to 24 hours. Store at room temperature, away from heat and light; use within 1 year.

To use, massage a dab of the balm into your feet, hands, shins, elbows, knees, or anywhere your skin is extremely dry, at least twice daily to condition your skin. The best time to apply it is immediately following a shower or bath, when your skin is still slightly damp.

Note: Safe for folks 2 years of age and older; for children under 2 or if pregnant or breastfeeding, omit the myrrh essential oil

Hammertoes

When ligaments and tendons tighten and force a toe to curl unnaturally, the toe can contract into a fixed position. In a hammertoe, both the joint at the ball of the foot and the joint at the end of the toe (the distal joint) bend upward, while the middle joint bends down. Hammertoes are the most common type of toe contraction, but there are two others: claw toes and mallet toes.

Claw toes also bend up at the joint at the ball of the foot, but bend down at both of the toe joints, resulting in an upside-down "U" or claw. Mallet toes bend down at just the distal joint, and the other two joints are normal. All three joint afflictions can affect any toe except the big one. They have the same causes and treatments.

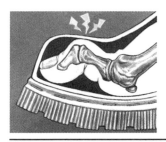

Hammertoe is often triggered by ill-fitting shoes.

Several factors are involved in the development of contracted toes. Wearing improper shoes that jam or compress the toes is a significant contributor. Faulty mechanics, such as a flat foot, high-arched foot, or Morton's toe, can be another big factor. Bunions can also force toes into abnormal positions, as can traumatic injury, birth defects, inflammatory arthritis, and neurological disorders resulting from diabetes and stroke. The risk of developing contracted toes increases with age.

Among people with contracted toes, some folks are asymptomatic, but most will experience some difficulty in moving their toes, as well as cramping, pain, swelling, redness, and difficulty wearing some kinds of shoes. Calluses and corns may develop on top of the raised or protruding joint and may evolve into open wounds or ulcers if sufficiently irritated.

TREATMENT Wear shoes with soft uppers, a high and broad toe box, a flat or minimal heel of ½ inch or less, and a good ½ inch of extra space beyond the tips of your toes. This should be your first treatment consideration, as it allows additional room for the other toes and less friction between them.

To moderate the pain of contracted toes, you can try products such as hammertoe cushions or pads, gel toe shields, moleskin, or toe caps to cushion the toes. Toe separators such as YogaToes and Correct Toes will help straighten toes and increase the space between them. Also, be sure to tend to corns and calluses to reduce skin thickening and painful shoe friction.

Straps and splints made specially for hammertoes (or, more specifically, hammertoes with some flexibility) can be used to hold the toe in a straight position, which will reduce pressure from shoes. And be sure to perform foot exercises daily to stretch and strengthen the feet (see Chapter 2). Taking yoga classes that target feet strength and flexibility can also aid in stretching and relaxing the foot's connective tissues.

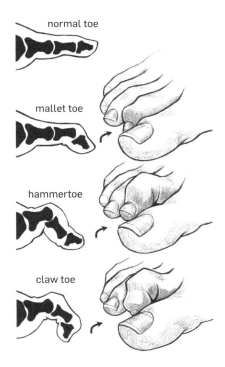

normal toe

mallet toe

hammertoe

claw toe

PREVENTION Unless your contracted toes are congenital or due to an injury or disease, the main prevention is wearing shoes that truly fit, doing foot exercises on a consistent basis, and going barefoot as often as possible. Keep your feet flexible and healthy!

MEDICAL ADVICE If your hammertoe, claw toe, or mallet toe problems persist, even though you are wearing properly fitted shoes and attempting the other treatments suggested above, corrective surgery may be an option, but it should be your last consideration. Talk to your podiatrist about the best approach. Chiropractors, osteopaths, and physical therapists who specialize in extremity realignment or sports rehabilitation may be able to help as well.

Heel Spurs

Heel spurs (or calcaneal spurs) occur at the attachment of the plantar fascia ligament to the heel bone. These small, pointed, bony growths, visible on an X-ray, begin to form when microtears of the plantar fascia ligament cause inflammation, swelling, tenderness, and sometimes bleeding. The stress results in calcium deposits, which slowly build up over time. It's not the spur that causes heel pain, it's the inflammation of the ligament pulling on the spur and the associated soft tissue injury and nerve irritation.

Heel spurs can be triggered by obesity, prolonged athletic activities, trauma to the heel, standing on your feet all day, improper footwear (especially high heels), pregnancy, Achilles tendonitis, flat feet, excessively high arches, and biomechanical imbalances. Anything that repeatedly strains or tears the plantar fascia and irritates the surrounding soft tissues can lead to the formation of a spur. Heel spurs are most common in women and senior folks.

A heel spur can feel like you have a small stone permanently wedged in your heel or like a painful bruise or throbbing ache. The pain is most intense immediately after a period of rest, such as when you are waking up, and can morph into a dull ache throughout the rest of the day. At times, the more you walk, the better your foot feels, up to a point. Continued walking and long periods of standing will cause the heel to become quite tender. Some folks can have a heel spur and not even be aware it's there. Everyone is different.

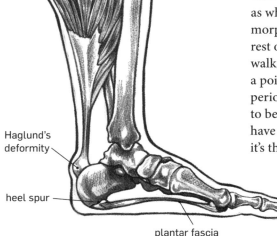

Haglund's deformity

heel spur

plantar fascia

TREATMENT Rest, ice, and elevation are prescribed. Take a load off and elevate your foot several times per day. To relieve inflammation, apply an ice pack or frozen bag of veggies (wrapped in a thin towel to protect the skin) to the area for 10 to 20 minutes. Remove the ice for 15 minutes, then repeat.

While you are in pain, stop doing any form of exercise that requires pounding with your feet, even walking. Instead, focus on low-impact exercises such as yoga, Pilates, tai chi, gentle weight lifting, stretching, or working out on a rowing or elliptical machine.

Avoid walking in bare feet until you are pain-free, unless you are walking slowly on a very soft surface.

Always stretch your feet first thing in the morning and before any activity.

Stop wearing any shoes with heels over 1 inch.

Wear comfortable shoes that allow your toes to wiggle. Adding heel cushions made from foam or gel will help relieve pressure and absorb shock.

Sometimes removing the original insole and replacing it with a full-length gel insert helps.

Herbs that are natural anti-inflammatories and pain relievers, such as black pepper, cayenne, ginger, Indian frankincense, rosemary, and turmeric, can help, especially when consumed as a blended supplement. They are a good alternative to NSAIDs (nonsteroidal anti-inflammatory drugs, such as aspirin and ibuprofen). Products containing these ingredients are usually found in the herbal pain-relief section of better natural foods stores, holistic pharmacies, and herb shops.

Feet need to be stretched and allowed to relax throughout the day. Several times a day, if possible, remove your shoes, point and flex your feet for as long as you can, and rotate your ankles. Calf stretches are advisable, too. Perform as many of the exercises in Chapter 2 as you can daily, to the best of your ability.

Another Pain in the Heel: Calcaneal Bumps

A calcaneal bump or Haglund's deformity (or "pump bump," as it is sometimes called) is a bony protuberance or enlargement on the upper back part of your heel where the Achilles tendon attaches to the bone. Women experience these far more than men.

The deformity is caused by increased friction on the heel by rubbing against hard, rigid heel counters—the portion of the shoe that adds stability for the heel. In most pump-style shoes, the heel counter is especially stiff, snug, and inflexible, which leads to irritation. Eventually a bursa sac (a fluid-filled "cushion") forms on the bump. This sac can then get inflamed and painful.

Changing your shoes to ones with a lower or softer heel counter or a heel counter that is notched for the Achilles tendon can help, as can icing the area, taking warm foot-baths with Epsom salts, and padding the bump with moleskin or foam.

PREVENTION

▸ Walk barefoot as often as you can and perform foot exercises and foot massage regularly, especially at the end of the day. This is essential to counter any damage inflicted by wearing ill-fitting shoes.

▸ When you do wear shoes, make sure they're comfortable. If you have a tendency to suffer from heel pain, find a shoe that gently cradles your heel and has ample heel padding, especially if your job demands that you be on your feet a great deal or you're an avid exerciser.

MEDICAL ADVICE If home therapies don't provide sufficient pain relief, a podiatrist may decide to try biomechanical taping or strapping or possibly custom orthotics in an attempt to redistribute your weight so that your foot is correctly balanced and the pressure is taken off the spur. Steroid injections are occasionally given for temporary relief. A chiropractor, osteopath, or physical therapist who specializes in extremity realignment or sports rehabilitation may also be able to help.

Hot Feet

There are some obvious causes of hot feet, such as walking barefoot on hot surfaces, wearing shoes and socks that are too heavy or that don't breathe, working outdoors in the heat, or standing all day in closed-toe shoes. Then there are medical conditions, such as high levels of stress and anxiety, pregnancy, hormone imbalances during menopause, hypothyroidism, high blood pressure, diabetic neuropathy, B vitamin deficiencies (folate, B_6, and B_{12}), Raynaud's disease, Grierson-Gopalan syndrome (burning feet syndrome), cardiovascular disease, and chemotherapy side effects, all of which often exhibit physical symptoms that include burning, tingling, numbness, and aching sensations in the feet (and hands).

Hot feet are generally not a serious threat to your health, just a nuisance. If your feet are hot, then usually so is the rest of you, and uncomfortable to boot! Frequently, the symptom of hot feet is combined with itchiness, profuse sweating, and/or odor, but we'll address those individually later. I just want to show you how you can bring basic relief to your fiery feet while cooling the rest of your body as well.

TREATMENT Try a cooling footbath. Add ½ cup of Epsom salts and 4 drops total of peppermint, lavender, and/or eucalyptus essential oils to a foot-soaking basin, then pour in enough cool/cold water to cover your feet up to your ankles. Soak for 10 to 20 minutes. Pat your feet dry, and follow with an application of your favorite foot cream or lotion (keep it in the refrigerator for extra cooling power). I recommend Peppermint-Lavender Foot Chiller (page 91) and Scent-sationally Cooling Aloe Foot Gel (page 92).

You could also elevate your bare feet and cover them with ice packs or frozen bags of veggies wrapped in a thin towel to protect your skin. Rest for 10 to 20 minutes. Ahhh . . .

FOOT NOTE
The average temperature inside your shoes is 106°F (41°C). It's a wonder your feet don't just sit down and go on strike!

Feet need fresh air, just like the rest of your body. Go barefoot as often as possible or wear open-toe shoes to avoid hot feet.

PREVENTION

▶ Wash your feet at least once but maybe twice a day with cool water, using a peppermint or tea tree essential oil soap. Don't forget to dry between your toes.

▶ Use a mint- or menthol-based foot powder liberally every morning and night to keep your feet delightfully dry and cool, or apply a light sprinkling of baking soda.

▶ Drink plenty of water—a dehydrated body produces more heat.

▶ Wear comfortable, roomy shoes with light, airy socks so your feet can breathe.

▶ If you must stand all day, remove your shoes every couple of hours and simply wiggle your toes and rotate your ankles for a bit of exercise.

MEDICAL ADVICE If your feet are not cooling down after using any of the simple remedies above, then a visit to your podiatrist or healthcare provider is called for to rule out a possible medical condition, nutritional deficiency, or medication side effect.

PEPPERMINT-LAVENDER FOOT CHILLER

YIELD

4 ounces

WHAT YOU NEED

16 drops peppermint essential oil

8 drops lavender essential oil

4-ounce dark glass spritzer bottle

½ cup unflavored vodka (80- or 100-proof)

½ teaspoon vegetable glycerin

Stimulating, refreshing relief is a quick spray away with this super-easy-to-make formula. Vodka and peppermint essential oil combine to form a menthol liniment of moderate intensity, with a cool-to-cold energy that evaporates rapidly, removing heat along with sweat and odor and leaving you feeling footloose and fancy-free. The lavender essential oil delivers comforting properties to stressed feet. I recommend stashing a small bottle in your gym bag to use as a postworkout foot refresher, especially if there's no time to shower—it'll put some spring back in your step!

Combine the essential oils in the spritzer bottle, then add the vodka and glycerin. Screw the top on the bottle and shake vigorously to blend. Label, date, and set the bottle in a cool, dark location for 24 hours so the spray can synergize. Store at room temperature, away from heat and light; use within 2 years.

Shake the bottle well before each use. Spray on your bare feet whenever they're feeling hot and tired. Allow your feet to air-dry before putting on socks or hosiery.

Note: Safe for folks 6 years of age and older; if pregnant or breastfeeding, replace the peppermint essential oil with lemon or grapefruit essential oil

YIELD

1 treatment

WHAT YOU NEED

1 tablespoon chilled
  aloe vera gel

2 drops peppermint
  essential oil

2 drops rosemary
  essential oil

SCENT-SATIONALLY COOLING ALOE FOOT GEL

This lovely gel smells fresh and uplifting as it delivers a most bracing experience to your hot feet! Pleasingly aromatic rosemary and peppermint essential oils combined with the cooling energy of aloe vera gel will comfort, chill, deodorize, and hydrate skin tissue, resulting in smiling feet.

Mix all the ingredients thoroughly in a very small bowl. Using light, brisk, gliding strokes, quickly massage the blend into your feet and lower legs. Deep, slow massage strokes will generate heat, which is not what you want. Allow it to soak into your skin for 5 minutes or so.

When you're finished, wipe any excess gel from your feet, or don a pair of socks and let it all soak in.

Note: Safe for folks 12 years of age or older; for children aged 6–11, reduce the essential oils by half; if pregnant or breastfeeding, replace the rosemary and peppermint essential oils with grapefruit, lavender, and/or lemon essential oils

Call the Experts

While many common foot ailments can be addressed with a change in footwear, regular exercises, and homemade herbal remedies, any condition that does not respond to home treatment is cause for medical attention. In my discussion of each ailment, I point out when medical care is warranted and suggest that you consult one or more of these professionals.

CERTIFIED FOOT CARE NURSE A foot care nurse does nursing assessments; performs nail cutting; treats calluses, dry skin, and infection; and provides information and support to assist patients with maintaining healthy feet. Many work alongside podiatrists or in hospitals and clinics, often with seniors or patients with diabetes, dementia, or arthritis who have difficulty caring for their feet or have special medical needs.

CHIROPRACTOR A doctor of chiropractic (DC) focuses on treatment through manual adjustment and/or manipulation of the spine. Chiropractic adjustments of your feet—and elsewhere in your body, as required—can help improve function, relieve pain, and protect against disorders stemming from or causing foot problems.

HEALTHCARE PROVIDER Also known as your primary care physician (PCP), this medical professional can diagnose and treat common foot problems or refer you to a specialist if necessary.

OSTEOPATH A doctor of osteopathy (DO) is a licensed physician who practices medicine using both conventional treatments and osteopathic manipulations to relieve pain and tension in the body. Treatment may also include stretching and advice on home exercises and proper shoes. In addition to treating the foot and ankle directly, they may work on the knees, hips, pelvis, and back, as needed.

PODIATRIST A doctor of podiatric medicine (DPM) is a surgeon who treats the foot, ankle, and related structures of the leg. They may specialize in a field such as sports medicine or diabetic care.

PHYSICAL THERAPIST Most physical therapists have attained a doctorate in physical therapy (DPT). They play an important role in preventive care and pain management, as well as overseeing rehabilitation and treatment for postsurgical patients and individuals with chronic ailments. When addressing issues of the feet, a physical therapist may work on functions such as gait (how you walk), how your body bears weight, balance, and mobility.

Ingrown Toenails

This common and painful ailment affects millions of folks every year, especially teens and seniors. Most often involving the big toe, it happens when the edge or corner of the nail turns under and digs into the skin. In response, the skin at the site becomes irritated and tender, with minor swelling, accompanied by pain when pressure is placed on the toe. Fluid may accumulate around the toenail.

If the nail edge breaks the skin, bacterial infection may arise, initiating additional symptoms, including increased swelling and extreme pain, bleeding, and the formation of pus. Walking may become unbearable. The risk of complications is higher with diabetes or other medical conditions that cause poor circulation.

You may tend toward ingrown toenails if you have an irregularly shaped, curved toenail or a small nail surrounded by an unusually large fleshy area, but they are frequently caused by cutting the toenails too short and rounding the nail edges. Wearing ill-fitting shoes that are too narrow or short or wearing tight socks or hosiery that press the nail edges into the fleshy

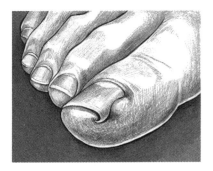

portion of the toe can trigger the problem, as can trauma such as stubbing or jamming your toe, dropping something heavy on your foot, or kicking a ball repeatedly.

Obese individuals are particularly susceptible because feet gain weight just like the rest of the body, and with the extra weight, the skin can swell up and around the toenail. Combine this with excess pressure placed upon the feet and a bit of improper nail clipping, and you have the perfect recipe for an ingrown toenail and infection. Older folks may also be at higher risk because their toenails tend to thicken with age, and they are sometimes unable to perform proper, regular foot care.

TREATMENT To provide pain relief in the early stages, soak your affected toe in a strong tea made with dried sage and salt. To make it, bring 1 gallon of water (or more, depending on the size of your foot-soaking basin) to a boil, add ½ cup of dried sage leaves, and remove from the heat. Cover and let steep for 20 minutes, then strain and let cool to a comfortable temperature. Pour the tea into the basin; you need just enough tea to cover the top of your foot. Add ½ cup of sea salt or Epsom salts and stir to dissolve. Soak your foot for 20 minutes. Dry thoroughly. Place a drop of tea tree or lavender essential oil or a dab of topical antibiotic ointment directly on the affected area to help keep infection at bay. Repeat the soak in this chapter two or three times per day until the pain is relieved. For a simpler, though still effective, soak, you may omit the sage leaves.

If the affected toenail is too short, don't try cutting it any further. Sharp instruments such as toenail nippers must be used with utmost care. Poking into irritated flesh while trying to cut away the offending nail edge can worsen the situation and trigger infection. Allow the nail to grow just past the tip of the toe before cutting it straight across.

Ingrown toenail pain reliever gel, available at drugstores and pharmacies, contains 1 percent sodium sulfide for pain relief, plus ingredients that soften the nail for easier trimming. This product really soothes an uncomfortable situation. To avoid further trauma to an ingrown toenail, avoid wearing tight-fitting footwear.

PREVENTION

- Always clip toenails straight across so that they are just about even with the tip of the toe and file smooth.
- Do not rip off broken or ragged toenails by hand. This results in jagged edges and hooks that can pierce the skin as the nail grows.
- Always wear comfortable shoes, socks, and hosiery. Remember— toes need wiggle room.

MEDICAL ADVICE If home care hasn't helped reduce symptoms after 3 to 5 days, the pain is worsening, and you find it difficult to walk or perform other activities, a visit to a certified foot care nurse, podiatrist, or healthcare provider is in order. If you're diabetic, don't allow a minor foot malady to become potentially life-threatening—seek immediate treatment.

For an infection, antibiotics (oral and/or topical) may be prescribed. If an ingrown toenail is a recurrent problem, your doctor may recommend minor surgery to remove a portion of the ingrown toenail. The procedure also helps prevent the offending nail portion from returning.

Itchy Feet

Itchy feet can have myriad causes, including athlete's foot, toenail fungus, scabies (mites), bug bites, underactive thyroid, eczema, psoriasis, diabetes, simple dry skin, iron deficiency anemia, essential fatty acid deficiency, pruritus gravidarum (severe itchiness in moms-to-be), and allergic contact dermatitis from exposure to poison ivy/oak or stinging nettle, a new detergent, or irritating sock fibers such as wool.

Itchy feet may feel hot and tingly, or dry and flaky, or inflamed. Sometimes they just need a good scratching because they've been confined in shoes all day and need fresh air. Unlike other spots, you can't scratch your feet every time you have the urge, which adds to the misery.

TREATMENT Remedies that cool and hydrate irritated skin are most beneficial. Menthol, a constituent derived from peppermint, has cooling, anti-itch, and deodorizing properties, which is why you often find peppermint or menthol in foot care products. You can make your own remedy by adding 12 drops of peppermint essential oil to 1 ounce (2 tablespoons) of your favorite natural lotion, cream, or oil. Stir to blend. Apply as needed. (**Caution:** For use with children 6 to 11 years old, reduce the essential oil by half. If pregnant or breastfeeding, avoid peppermint essential oil and substitute lavender or geranium essential oil.) Or try my Mineral-Rich Oatmeal Soak recipe (page 82), which works wonders for dry, itchy feet.

Try wrapping your itchy feet with cold, damp towels for 15 minutes, or surround them with bags of frozen veggies or ice packs, being sure to place a thin towel between your skin and the frozen items.

When I have itchy skin, my go-to homeopathic remedy is Ledum Palustre 30c by Boiron. These tiny tablets work quite well to relieve itchiness anywhere on the body from bug bites, dermatitis, hives, rashes, and so on, plus they comfort stiffness, achiness, and swelling of joints.

Apple cider vinegar is a traditional remedy for itchy feet. Baking soda is another. Add 1 cup of apple cider vinegar or ½ cup of baking soda to a foot-soaking basin filled ankle-deep with cool water. Soak your feet for 15 to 20 minutes. Pat dry, then apply a peppermint-based foot cream or oil or a thin layer of chilled aloe vera juice or gel. Note: Avoid the vinegar soak if your feet are deeply cracked, bleeding, or extremely inflamed, as it will sting like heck!

PREVENTION

▸ Wear 100 percent cotton socks, or at least ones with a high percentage of cotton. Cashmere-cotton socks are lovely in winter. Hemp socks are soft and quite durable. Wool socks are notoriously irritating to sensitive skin.

▸ Moisturize your feet daily. The soles of the feet contain no oil glands and can lose elasticity and moisture, which results in dry skin and cracking. Dry skin itches!

▸ Eat a healthy, whole-foods diet with ample skin-nourishing fats, such as those in grass-fed butter, extra-virgin olive oil, sesame oil, avocados (and their oil), raw nuts and seeds (and butters made from them), and fatty fish such as salmon, sardines, tuna, and kippers.

▸ Apply a natural foot powder to your feet every day to keep itchy fungus at bay. Try the Fungus Fighter Foot Powder recipe on page 58.

MEDICAL ADVICE If the above treatments fail and the itchiness persists longer than 2 weeks, it progresses further up your leg, or an unusual rash, burning sensation, or swelling appears, please pay a visit to your podiatrist or healthcare provider, as they may want to rule out a fungal infection, other skin disease, or an underlying medical condition.

YIELD

1 ounce

WHAT YOU NEED

2 tablespoons calendula-infused oil

3 drops Roman chamomile essential oil

3 drops tea tree essential oil

1-ounce dark glass bottle with dropper top

SOOTHING ANTI-ITCH OIL

Calendula-infused oil (available from holistic pharmacies, natural foods stores, and herb shops) has vulnerary properties (meaning it soothes, cools, and helps mend skin). It is an especially effective anti-itch remedy when combined with Roman chamomile and tea tree essential oils.

Combine the calendula oil and the essential oils in the bottle. Screw the top on the bottle and shake well to blend. Label and date the bottle, and set it in a cool, dark location for 24 hours so that the oils can synergize. Store at room temperature, away from heat and light; use within 1 year.

To use, wash your feet with soap and cool water. Dry. Massage approximately ½ teaspoon of the oil into each foot. When you're done, put on clean socks to encourage the oil to sink in.

Note: Safe for folks 6 years of age and older

Metatarsalgia

Metatarsalgia (met-uh-tahr-SAL-gee-a) is a condition in which the ball of the foot, where the heads of the metatarsal bones meet the toes, becomes inflamed, bruised, and quite uncomfortable when bearing weight. It can be caused by wearing shoes with high heels, even as low as 1 inch, which puts added pressure on the five metatarsal heads. Shoes that are too narrow or too tapered to allow full mobility of the forefoot and even weight distribution on the metatarsal heads can also be a problem, forcing one or more of the metatarsals

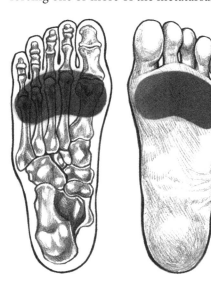

to drop out of alignment. High-arched feet, hammertoes, bunions, Morton's neuroma, Morton's toe, inflammatory arthritis, thin feet without much fat padding and with prominent bones, being overweight, and participating in high-impact activities in shoes that don't fit properly can contribute to metatarsalgia.

Anything that causes you to come down hard on your metatarsals can lead to pain in this area. Even a previous foot surgery or stress fracture that has altered the shape of your foot can contribute to increased loading on the ball of the foot.

With metatarsalgia, you may experience sharp or aching pain or burning sensations that worsen when you stand, run, jump, flex your feet, or walk, especially barefoot on a hard surface, but improve when you rest. Some folks say it feels like they've got a pebble in their shoe or a bone bruise. You may experience sharp or shooting pain, numbness, or tingling sensations in your toes. Calluses may develop due to excessive pressure in the affected area. Though generally not serious, metatarsalgia can definitely sideline you.

TREATMENT Take a load off for a few days. Keep your problem foot elevated as much as possible. Icing the affected area for 20 minutes several times per day can be helpful to reduce inflammation, especially in the first 24 to 48 hours.

Herbs that are natural anti-inflammatories and pain relievers, such as black pepper, cayenne, ginger, Indian frankincense, rosemary, and turmeric, can help, especially when consumed as a blended supplement. They are a good alternative to NSAIDs (nonsteroidal anti-inflammatory drugs, such as aspirin and ibuprofen). Products containing these ingredients are usually found in the herbal pain-relief section of better natural foods stores, holistic pharmacies, and herb shops.

Shoes must have a wide toe box. No binding or squeezing of the metatarsals is allowed. A cushioned metatarsal pad placed under the metatarsal heads of the forefoot can often provide much relief, as can full-length gel or foam inserts.

Start wearing toe separators, such as Correct Toes or YogaToes, to improve the spacing between your toes and metatarsals and the realignment of your feet. Begin slowly, and gradually increase the time for which you can wear these devices without too much discomfort.

If you are a runner/jogger/walker, reduce your mileage and exercise on softer surfaces, or switch to a lower-impact activity.

Strengthen your forefoot by performing daily foot exercises. Do as many of the exercises in Chapter 2 as you can, as often as you can. The Toe Spread exercise (page 25) is especially recommended.

Foot massage can help relieve pain and swelling and relax tight foot muscles. Use the techniques in Chapter 3 (or ask someone to massage your feet) on a daily basis. Try the Step Lively Massage Oil (page 102), which can provide blessed relief to achy feet, especially when applied daily.

Schedule a few appointments with a foot reflexologist or massage therapist for a focused relaxation session to ease tension and tightness in your feet and lower legs.

PREVENTION

▸ Wear flat-soled, foot-shaped shoes with a wide toe box, and go barefoot as often as you can so your metatarsals can splay.

▸ If you're an avid exerciser, please wear shoes that provide a bit of cushioning—but not excessive cushioning—between you and the pavement. No "barefoot shoes," please, unless your feet are super strong and conditioned for exercising in this minimalist form of footwear.

▸ Keep your feet strong and flexible by doing foot exercises, calf stretches, and foot massage regularly.

MEDICAL ADVICE If changing shoe styles and attempting the treatments above fail to provide sufficient relief, contact your podiatrist, chiropractor, or osteopath. Left untreated, metatarsalgia may alter your gait due to limping, leading to pain in other parts of the same or opposite foot and pain elsewhere in the body, such as the lower back or hip.

YIELD

2 ounces

WHAT YOU NEED

8 drops copaiba essential oil

8 drops peppermint essential oil

8 drops Roman chamomile essential oil

2-ounce dark glass bottle with a dropper top

¼ cup St. John's wort–infused oil

STEP LIVELY MASSAGE OIL

With its beautiful reddish hue, this oil blend delivers a cooling energy and refreshing relief to dog-tired feet. It helps reduce inflammation and pain while adding a bit of spring to your step—perfect after running, walking, hiking, doing chores, or a long day at work or chasing after kids.

Combine the essential oils in the bottle, then add the St. John's wort oil. Screw the top on the bottle and shake vigorously for 2 minutes to blend. Label and date the bottle and set it in a cool, dark location for 24 hours so that the oils can synergize. Store at room temperature, away from heat and light; use within 1 year.

Shake well before each use. Massage 1–2 teaspoons into clean, dry feet, ankles, and calves, using as much pressure as needed to alleviate fatigue and tension. When you're finished, wipe any excess oil from your feet, or don a pair of socks and let it all soak in.

BONUS USE: This oil is a most wonderful aid to ease the pain of bruised tissue in your feet, ankles, or legs following an injury. Gently massage a few drops into the affected area up to three times daily until the bruise fades.

Note: Safe for folks 12 years of age and older; for children aged 6–11, reduce the essential oils by half; for children aged 2–5, use just plain St. John's wort–infused oil; if pregnant or breastfeeding, replace the peppermint essential oil with grapefruit or lemon essential oil

Morton's Neuroma

Also called an intermetatarsal neuroma or a forefoot neuroma, this condition was first described in 1876 by Dr. Thomas George Morton. It is associated with nerve inflammation and thickening of the surrounding tissue, which causes pain and results from long-term pressure from injury, ongoing irritation, or compression of one of the plantar digital nerves that supplies sensation to the toes. This neuroma typically affects the area between the third and fourth toes and the portion of the ball of the foot immediately below, but occasionally the second and third toes.

Activities that transmit repetitive forces to the ball of the foot, such as running, tap dancing, and racquet sports, and wearing high heels and narrow- or tapered-toe shoes—anything that causes the nerves between the toes and metatarsal heads to become stretched, rubbed, or compressed—can trigger the growth of a neuroma. Folks with bunions, hammertoes, high arches, and flat feet are also more prone to this malady.

When you have Morton's neuroma, you'll often experience burning, shooting, stabbing pain and/or tingling and numbness between the toes and in the ball of the foot. Sometimes it feels like you've stepped on a pebble or small marble. The pain and discomfort can come and go. Once again, this problem most often affects women who wear binding shoe styles. The symptoms may begin gradually and occur only occasionally, when you're wearing narrow shoes or performing certain aggravating activities, but over time symptoms can progressively worsen and persist for days or weeks. If not remedied, symptoms become more intense as the neuroma enlarges.

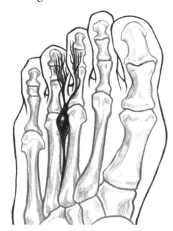

The inflamed nerve radiates pain between the toes and in the ball of the foot.

TREATMENT When you feel pain in this region of your forefoot, promptly remove your shoe and massage your foot. Relieving your foot of shoe compression often brings quick relief. Of course, the pain *will* keep coming back if you squeeze your feet back into those shoes, and if left untreated, it can become excruciating, so much so that walking becomes unbearable. It can also lead to permanent nerve damage in the affected area. I recommend the same treatments suggested for metatarsalgia (page 100).

PREVENTION Though it's not always possible to prevent Morton's neuroma, you can greatly reduce your risk by wearing comfortable shoes that truly fit with minimal or no heel elevation and plenty of wiggle room for your toes. Also, keep your feet strong and flexible by doing the foot exercises in Chapter 2

daily—the Toe Spread exercise (page 25) is especially valuable to increase the space between your toes and metatarsals to prevent potential entrapment of the intermetatarsal nerves.

MEDICAL ADVICE Home treatments can bring significant relief, but if you're not responding as well as you'd like, please schedule a visit to your podiatrist. During your exam, your doctor will press on your foot to feel for a tender spot or mass or a clicking between the metatarsal heads. An MRI or ultrasound can confirm the diagnosis. Most podiatrists prefer that patients exhaust all treatment options, such as cushioning orthotics, physical therapy, or pain-relieving injections, before suggesting surgery. Though usually effective, surgery can result in permanent numbness of the affected toes.

Morton's Toe

In folks with Morton's toe, the first metatarsal bone (the long bone in line with your big toe) is shorter than normal and makes the second toe appear abnormally long. Also called Morton's foot, Morton's syndrome, Greek foot, or royal toe, this relatively common anatomical arrangement was identified in the 1930s by Dr. Dudley J. Morton. For once, I'm not going to blame this condition on shoes. Instead, blame your parents. It's hereditary, like most features of your bone structure.

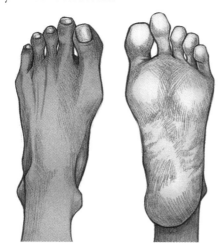

It's not uncommon to have a big toe that is shorter than the second toe.

Under normal conditions, when you run and walk, the spring muscles of the big toe and medial arch push the foot off the ground with each step, but with a case of Morton's toe, the big toe can't perform its job as well as it should. Because it provides less than adequate support for the foot during each step, the second toe, which is naturally weaker, has to carry more of the weight, leading to ligament disruption. This causes a weight shift, which can potentially lead to biomechanical issues affecting the ankle, knee, hip, and lower back.

Morton's toe causes pain to develop in the ball of the foot (and therefore is one of the many possible causes of metatarsalgia), often because the base of the second metatarsal becomes inflamed and can be accompanied by medial arch fatigue. Pain usually arises with walking or standing and improves with rest. Toenail trauma is common.

If a subungual hematoma (blood beneath the nail) develops, the nail will change color and may fall off. The constant pressure that walking and standing place on the longer second toe can lead to callus formation under the second and third metatarsal heads.

Additionally, because the tip of the second toe tends to push against the end of the shoe (which is usually too short to accommodate the toe), the tendons and ligaments that control that toe may become contracted and imbalanced, leading to a hammertoe deformity, with the development of a corn on top and a blister on the tip of the toe.

TREATMENT Any pain caused by Morton's toe can usually be resolved with home treatment. Sometimes it's as simple as wearing shoes with a high and wide toe box and going up half a size to accommodate the longer toe. Replacing the insoles in your shoes with ones made of a nonslippery material will keep your foot from sliding forward. A cushioned metatarsal pad placed under the metatarsal heads of the forefoot can often relieve pain and pressure on the second metatarsal head by adding support to the shaft of the second metatarsal bone.

To treat issues commonly associated with Morton's toe, such as calluses, corns, blisters, hammertoes, and metatarsal pain/metatarsalgia, refer to the individual treatment suggestions in this chapter.

PREVENTION Since Morton's toe is a genetic gift from Mother Nature, you can't prevent it like you can other afflictions. The key is to make your foot comfortable and help prevent the secondary problems from occurring.

MEDICAL ADVICE For help with unrelenting pain, a podiatrist might suggest physical therapy, plus specific foot exercises, and perhaps custom orthotics to ease discomfort and help prevent the degenerative changes that can result from improper alignment. As a last resort, surgery may be recommended.

Odoriferous and Sweaty Feet

One of our skin's important functions is to regulate our body temperature. The body loses the most heat via the head, armpits, hands, and feet. In fact, there are more sweat glands per square inch in the soles of the feet than on any other part of the body. Enclosed shoes, whatever material they are made of, often accumulate sweat. The lack of ventilation, plus the fairly common combination of moisture, heat, and poor hygiene, can cause the top layer of skin on the feet to soften and break down.

It's not the sweat that causes the odor but the bacteria that normally reside on the feet feeding off the sweat and skin debris. Fungi also thrive in moist, warm environments and can cause odor.

Though rarely a health issue, foot odor (the medical term is plantar bromhidrosis) can be seriously embarrassing. The rate of sweat production is greatly affected by emotions such as fear, nervousness, and stress.

Additionally, exercising heavily, working at a physically demanding job, becoming overheated, or standing for extended periods of time will also cause the feet to sweat. Being overweight is associated with increased sweating. Some folks have a genetic predisposition to foot odor and wetness.

Foot odor can be described as musty, cheesy, rancid . . . whatever the adjective, this rather distinctive aroma can permeate an entire room when the affected individual removes their shoes. Excessive perspiration will lead to rapid deterioration of footwear; the materials break down prematurely from the day-to-day pressure combined with constant moisture.

TREATMENT In addition to following the suggested daily foot care routine on page 12, be sure not to wear the same pair of closed-toe shoes on consecutive days. Always allow a pair of shoes to dry for 24 hours before wearing them again.

FOOT NOTE
A pair of feet contain approximately 250,000 sweat glands, which can release about 8 ounces of moisture each day!

A Remedy for Smelly Shoes

Fill a pair of thin cotton socks with baking soda (about ½ cup per sock) and close off the opening with a rubber band. Insert a sock into each shoe, spreading it out from toe to heel, and leave for 24 hours. Your shoes will smell much fresher after this treatment, guaranteed. You can dry out and reuse the "soda socks" several times before replacing the baking soda.

PREVENTION

- Wear insoles impregnated with baking soda or charcoal in your shoes, and change them often.
- Spritz or wipe 70 percent isopropyl (rubbing) alcohol onto the bottom of your feet if they get sweaty often. Allow to air-dry. The alcohol kills bacteria and rapidly evaporates away stench. You can do this two or three times a day as a preventive measure or use it as a quick fix for stinky feet.
- Some folks find that applying antiperspirant to their feet is effective in reducing sweat and odor. Or try an herbal deodorant; it may not lessen sweat and prevent bacterial growth, but it will help reduce odor.
- If you're prone to foot odor, minimize your consumption of sulfur-containing foods such as garlic, onions, mustard and turnip greens, kale, and eggs. Also avoid certain moldy cheeses and heavily yeasted foods such as beer and sourdough breads.
- Increase your intake of chlorophyll, which is a known internal-odor fighter. Spirulina, chlorella, parsley, wheat/barley grass, and green drinks are high in chlorophyll.

MEDICAL ADVICE The above recommendations will often produce positive results, but if they don't, please contact your podiatrist or healthcare provider for a thorough checkup. Medical conditions such as hyperhidrosis, hyperthyroidism, adrenal insufficiency, chronic anxiety/panic attacks, Parkinson's disease, and hormonal imbalances can cause profuse sweating, as can alcoholism and obesity. You don't need to suffer or feel self-conscious due to foot odor. There is a solution.

FRESHEN-UP FOOT SOAP

This liquid soap gently cleans and disinfects sweaty, smelly feet and effectively removes odor-causing bacteria without overdrying the skin. It's helpful for keeping foot and toenail fungus at bay, too. I often use this blend to wash the feet of my reflexology clients prior to treatment.

YIELD

16 ounces

WHAT YOU NEED

- 12 drops lemon essential oil
- 12 drops peppermint essential oil
- 12 drops tea tree essential oil
- 12 drops thyme essential oil
- 1 (16-ounce) bottle liquid castile soap, peppermint or unscented

Add the essential oils directly to the bottle of castile soap. Screw the top on the bottle and shake vigorously to blend. Store the finished product right in the bottle, or decant it into smaller storage containers, preferably plastic squeeze bottles, if desired. Label and date. Store in a dark, cool cabinet or in the shower; use within 1 year.

Shake well before each use. It's very concentrated, so a little goes a long, long way! Add a squirt or two to a footbath of warm water or use in the shower. Wash feet twice daily. Afterward, thoroughly dry with a towel, then follow with an application of your favorite foot powder.

Note: Safe for folks 2 years of age and older; if pregnant or breastfeeding, replace the peppermint and thyme essential oils with lemon, tea tree, lavender, or sweet orange essential oils

FEELIN' FRESH CLEANSING FOOT SPRAY

Witch hazel extract, valued for its astringent, tissue-tightening properties, is the perfect base for this foot spritzer. With the cooling, refreshing, deodorizing, and antimicrobial properties of the essential oils, it's the perfect blend to help combat smelly feet, especially when a footbath isn't possible.

YIELD

4 ounces

WHAT YOU NEED

- 6 drops lavender essential oil
- 6 drops lemon essential oil
- 6 drops peppermint essential oil
- 6 drops tea tree essential oil
- 4-ounce dark glass spritzer bottle
- ½ cup witch hazel extract

Add the essential oils directly to the spritzer bottle, then pour in the witch hazel. Screw the top on the bottle and shake vigorously to blend. Label and date the bottle. Store at room temperature, away from heat and light; use within 1 year.

Shake well before each use. Spray on your bare feet whenever they're feeling particularly sweaty or stinky, wipe with a towel, and then spray again. Allow your feet to air-dry before putting on socks or hosiery.

Note: Safe for folks 6 years of age and older; if pregnant or breastfeeding, replace the peppermint essential oil with additional lavender, lemon, or tea tree essential oil

2 cups

ODOR-NEUTRALIZING HERBAL FOOT POWDER

A very effective deodorizing foot (and underarm) powder, indeed! The peppermint essential oil delivers a punch of cooling, refreshing menthol, while the lemon, tea tree, and thyme essential oils bring antiseptic properties and a superb ability to eliminate foot stench and keep it at bay. Zinc oxide powder (available from pharmacies and online cosmetic ingredient suppliers) works as a natural astringent antiperspirant and also minimizes bacterial proliferation.

WHAT YOU NEED

1 cup baking soda

½ cup cornstarch or arrowroot powder

½ cup white cosmetic clay (also known as powdered white clay or kaolin)

1 tablespoon zinc oxide powder

50 drops peppermint essential oil

30 drops lemon essential oil

10 drops tea tree essential oil

10 drops thyme essential oil

Shaker containers (glass, plastic, or cardboard)

1 Combine the baking soda, cornstarch, white clay, and zinc oxide in a medium bowl and gently mix with a whisk. Add the essential oils a few drops at a time, whisking them in as you go. (You can also pulse the dry ingredients in a food processor and continue pulsing as you add the essential oils.)

2 Transfer the powder to an airtight container and store in a dark, cool place for 3 days to allow the essential oils' fragrance and remedial properties to permeate the mixture.

3 Package the blend in small shaker containers. Label and date. Store at room temperature, away from heat and light; use within 1 year.

To use, sprinkle the powder into your socks once or twice daily, or apply to dry, bare feet.

Note: Safe for folks 6 years of age and older; if pregnant or breastfeeding, replace the peppermint and thyme essential oils with lemon, tea tree, lavender, or sweet orange essential oil

Plantar Fasciitis

The plantar fascia is a thick band of fibrous connective tissue that runs from the heel bone to the base of the toes, supporting the foot's arches and functioning as a shock absorber. Fasciitis is inflammation resulting from strain, with microtears within the tissue. Factors that lead to plantar fasciitis include having calf muscles so tight that it is difficult to dorsiflex the foot (pull it back toward the shin), obesity, having either a very high arch or a flat foot, repetitive impact activities, or new or increased physical activity. A sudden change in footwear, such as going from heels to flats or vice versa, may stress the plantar fascia, as can spending a lot of time on your feet.

Inflammation is the body's natural response to injury, and in this case it results in aching, throbbing, burning, or stabbing pain on the inside or medial edge and/or center of the heel, which tends to be worse upon arising from sleep or prolonged rest and lessens with activity, but as the day progresses, it usually returns with a vengeance. Pain may also radiate into the medial arch.

The plantar fascia has poor circulation, so it is slow to heal and can be quite stiff. At times, plantar fasciitis seemingly develops without any reason, and strangely enough, the pain can be intermittent.

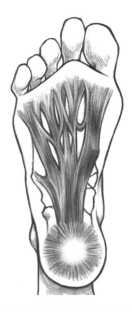

The focal point of pain from plantar fasciitis is most often felt in the heel.

TREATMENT Simple home treatments will often provide significant relief from your misery within 6 weeks or so, but be aware that it can take much longer. Be consistent and have patience.

First and foremost, stop all impact activities for as long as you're feeling any pain in your foot, which may be several weeks or even months. Your foot needs time to heal. Try low- or no-impact activities such as tai chi, yoga, Pilates, swimming, stationary weight training, using an elliptical trainer, rowing, and so on.

Postactivity, elevate your affected foot and chill it for 10 to 20 minutes with an ice pack or frozen bag of corn or peas wrapped with a thin towel to protect your skin. Remove the ice for 15 minutes, then repeat. Do this several times per day. Alternatively, you can roll your foot over a frozen water bottle for 10 minutes, three times per day.

Stop wearing any shoe with a heel higher than 1 inch. While your foot is healing, always wear shoes with some cushioning. Insert silicone, gel, or foam heel cushions to provide extra shock absorption in the heel area. Full-length gel or foam insoles can also deliver pain relief. Avoid going barefoot unless you are walking slowly on a very soft surface.

Perform exercises that loosen, stretch, and strengthen your feet and calves. Chapter 2 has a good variety; do as many of the exercises as you can, every day.

Foot massage can help relieve pain and swelling and relax tight fascia and muscles. See Chapter 3 for some good techniques and perform all of them yourself (or ask someone to do them for you) on a daily basis. Try the Step Lively Massage Oil recipe on page 102—when applied daily, it provides blessed relief to achy feet.

Schedule a few appointments with a foot reflexologist or massage therapist for a focused relaxation session to ease tension and tightness in your feet and lower legs.

Herbs that are natural anti-inflammatories and pain relievers, such as black pepper, cayenne, ginger, Indian frankincense, rosemary, and turmeric, can help, especially when consumed as a blended supplement. They are a good alternative to NSAIDs (nonsteroidal anti-inflammatory drugs, such as aspirin and ibuprofen). Products containing these ingredients are usually found in the herbal pain-relief section of better natural foods stores, holistic pharmacies, and herb shops.

PREVENTION

- Always stretch feet first thing in the morning or before any activity.
- Do your foot exercises regularly to keep your feet and calves strong and flexible.
- Maintain a healthy body weight.
- Wear flexible shoes that allow your feet to move and stretch fully as they should. Minimize your time in shoes with heels over 1 inch; this includes most athletic shoes, and any shoe in which the end of the toe box is elevated—look at the profile of the shoe to see if the sole lifts in the toe box area.
- If you have a tendency to suffer from heel pain or plantar fasciitis, find a shoe that gently cradles your heel and has ample heel padding, especially if your job demands that you be on your feet a great deal or you're an avid exerciser.

SEEK MEDICAL ADVICE If the pain becomes unbearable and you have difficulty walking in spite of consistent home care, consult a podiatrist. Recommendations might include physical therapy, stretching exercises, shock wave therapy, shoe modifications, foot taping or an arch brace, or a temporary custom orthotic. Plantar fasciitis can also result from a foot/ankle misalignment issue or biomechanical imbalances, which would need to be treated. Chiropractors, osteopaths, and physical therapists who specialize in extremity realignment or sports rehabilitation may be able to help.

FOOT NOTE

According to the American Podiatric Medical Association, "most Americans log an amazing 75,000 miles on their feet by the time they reach age 50."

Plantar Warts

Plantar warts, which develop on the plantar surface or sole of your foot, are caused by a strain of the human papilloma virus (HPV). You can easily transmit it to other parts of your body or to others, though not everyone who comes in contact with the virus will develop a wart. People with compromised immune systems are more likely to contract them. Once you have a wart, you are more likely to have another.

Just like the athlete's foot fungus, the virus that causes plantar warts can be contracted by walking barefoot in warm, moist environments, such as gyms, locker rooms, saunas, showers, pool areas, and public restrooms. Cracks or abrasions on your feet are an open invitation for the virus to take up residence. Scratching or shaving over the affected area can also spread

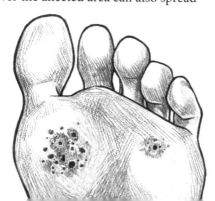

the infection, as can wearing poorly ventilated shoes that retain sweat and warmth.

Plantar warts are small, rough, granulated, spongy, and flat or ever-so-slightly raised growths or lesions, similar in texture to a cauliflower. They can appear singly or in multiples. You might sometimes mistake one for a corn that has become rough and scaly. A plantar wart, though, often has one or more teensy black dots in the center, which are blood vessels supplying the wart with nutrients and oxygen.

Warts can vary in color from white to pinkish, brownish, or dusty gray. They occur most frequently on the heels and balls of the feet and can penetrate deeply into the sole. They are typically quite tender, causing a great deal of discomfort when you stand or walk.

A mosaic wart, caused by the same virus, is irregular in shape and bleeds easily when irritated, and it can eventually form a large cluster of a hundred or more tiny warts. This patch of warts can cover the entire sole and has a rougher, thicker surface than a typical plantar wart.

TREATMENT The thick skin on the bottom of the foot makes plantar warts resistant to treatment. Thankfully, plantar warts generally are not a serious health concern and eventually disappear on their own, even without treatment. For a painful wart, however, there are a number of effective remedies that are worth trying. Keep in mind, however, that although warts can often be successfully eliminated, sometimes even aggressive medical intervention won't completely prevent their recurrence.

Duct tape. This "fix anything" tape removes the wart layer by layer. Just cover the wart with duct tape—use a piece big enough that it won't fall off easily. Every 4 to 6 days, remove the tape in the evening and soak your foot in warm water for 10 minutes or so to soften the skin. Dry thoroughly, then file the wart with an emery board or pumice stone to remove dead layers of skin (discard or disinfect your filing tool after use).

Allow your foot to dry and breathe overnight while you sleep. Reapply fresh tape in the morning. You have to be consistent to see results—it can take a couple of months to totally eradicate the wart.

Salicylic acid. Salicylic acid encourages the wart to peel and shed its tough layers. You can apply it, as an ointment or drops, directly to the wart, but please use with care. With repeated application, the acid can burn surrounding healthy skin and even cause an ulcer to form. The medicated disks, which are impregnated with salicylic acid, cushion the painful wart while simultaneously dissolving it. Always follow the manufacturer's directions.

Caution: Diabetics should never use salicylic acid products to treat their warts. Ulceration of the skin could lead to serious problems.

Herbal remedies. If the season is right and you can find these plants growing in your neighborhood, try applying the milky, sticky sap from a dandelion stem, calendula stem, or milkweed stem to the wart and covering it with an adhesive bandage. Change the dressing daily. These saps act as corrosive agents on the wart.

Tea tree essential oil, with its potent antiviral, antifungal, and antibacterial properties, can be effective in removing a wart. Simply apply 1 drop directly to the wart and cover it with a bandage. Repeat twice daily.

Apple cider vinegar. Soak a medium-size adhesive bandage with raw apple cider vinegar and apply it to your wart. The acetic acid will soften the tough tissue and encourage peeling. After 12 hours, remove the bandage, file the wart with an emery board or pumice stone (discard or disinfect your filing tool after use), and then reapply a fresh, soaked bandage. Do this twice daily for at least 30 days.

If you see no reduction in the size of the wart after about 30 days of any of these home treatments, try another treatment. Remember, no one treatment works for everyone. Whatever method you choose, keep at it. Warts can be stubborn.

PREVENTION

- Wash your hands carefully after touching a wart, whether it's on your own feet or someone else's.
- If you are prone to warts, don't share towels, bathmats, or shoes with anyone else, as the virus can transmit via shared personal items.
- Keep your feet clean and dry. Change your socks and shoes daily and replace your shoes if you have multiple recurrences of warts.

- Don't use the same emery board, pumice stone, or nail clipper on your warts as you use on your healthy skin and nails. Do not pick, scratch, or shave warts.
- Clean your shower/tub floor regularly with a 10 percent bleach solution or a commercial disinfectant to kill any resident viruses.
- Avoid walking barefoot in warm, moist, public environments such as in gyms, locker rooms, saunas, showers, and around swimming pools.

SEEK MEDICAL ADVICE If a plantar wart doesn't respond to home treatment, or begins to spread, bleed, change appearance or color, or otherwise become bothersome, or you aren't sure whether it really *is* a wart, see your healthcare provider or a podiatrist for an accurate diagnosis, ruling out the possibility that the skin lesion may actually be a type of skin cancer.

Medical treatments can include cryotherapy (freezing), chemical cautery (chemical application or injection), electrodessication (burning), laser surgery, or surgical excision. Try to avoid surgery, if possible, as it can be quite painful and result in scarring.

Toenail Fungus

Fungal infection is the most common disorder of the toenails, with the primary cause being dermatophytes, usually the same type that cause athlete's foot. These organisms are present pretty much everywhere: in your shoes, in communal showers, in locker rooms, around public pools, in saunas/steam rooms, and even in outdoor soil. They thrive in warm, dark, moist places. Various yeasts and molds can also cause nail infections. Whatever the cause, the result is unsightly and contagious, and it often causes its sufferers to avoid wearing open-toe shoes and any other situation that might call for bare feet.

Any weakness or trauma in the nail and surrounding tissues, including dry and cracked skin, psoriasis, eczema, or micro tissue injuries, provides a portal for the opportunistic fungi to enter. The infection is persistent because it lives within the nail bed, where it is difficult to reach and treat.

Toenail fungal infection often affects people who exercise regularly; all that pounding on the feet can result in nail trauma. It's more common in older adults and those with risk factors such as a weakened immune system and reduced blood circulation to the feet. Unlike athlete's foot, which can develop rapidly, nail infections tend to develop more slowly, after prolonged contact. They can start from an athlete's foot infection, and the reverse is also true—athlete's foot can result from a toenail fungal infection.

With the onset of infection, one or more of your toenails begins to look a bit abnormal. Color changes, such as long yellowish streaks or white or light brownish patches that can be scraped off, might appear. The nail may lift and begin to separate from the nail bed; it may thicken and become brittle and flaky. It can also become distorted in shape and begin to pit and twist.

TREATMENT AND PREVENTION
Please see the discussion of athlete's foot on page 54; much of the advice given there applies to toenail fungus as well.

SEEK MEDICAL ADVICE If allowed to progress, a toenail fungal infection can impact your general foot health, so if self-treatment is not remedying the infection, see a podiatrist, dermatologist, or your healthcare provider. They can prescribe topical or oral antifungal medications to use in conjunction with the above treatments and preventive measures. As with any medication, especially antifungal drugs, there are potential side effects, which can include liver toxicity—be aware of this and ask questions.

Don't be discouraged if your nail still looks disfigured even after 12 weeks of treatment. The nail plate can take a year or more to grow out fully, depending on age, circulation, and general health. Even when the fungus is completely eradicated, there may be long-term effects on the appearance of the nail.

YOUR FOOT CARE CUPBOARD

I recommend gathering your foot care supplies and keeping them in a basket or storage container for easy (and frequent!) access. You don't have to buy all the herbs and essential oils that I recommend here, but you'll find a brief explanation of which items you definitely need and which are nice to have for extra pampering.

Basic Equipment

To set yourself up for a decent home pedicure and for most of the herbal treatments, collect a few easy-to-obtain items, starting with a sturdy foot-soaking basin large enough to accommodate both feet and deep enough that you can fill it with enough water to cover your ankles. A plastic one is light, inexpensive, and easy to clean; I use a plastic dishwashing tub for personal use as well as for my foot reflexology practice. A stainless steel one is fine, too, but avoid aluminum or copper. Those metals might react with vinegar or Epsom salts.

Purchase some good-quality toenail clippers and a double-sided (one side coarse, one side fine) foot file or pediwand. Some people like pumice stones, but I find an implement with a handle easiest to use.

Some treatments call for a microwavable heating bag filled with flaxseed or rice or a small electric heating pad.

Finally, for making the simple recipes in this book, you'll need a few common kitchen utensils, such as a small mixing bowl, measuring spoons, and a couple of whisks (medium and small sizes). A miniature glass or stainless steel prep bowl is handy for mixing single treatments. You'll also need some containers for storing herbal preparations, such as shaker containers for powders, 2- and 4-ounce dark glass or plastic jars, 1- and 2-ounce dropper top bottles, and 4-ounce spray bottles.

You can obtain storage containers and the ingredients described below at natural foods stores or co-ops, better grocery stores and pharmacies, most herb shops, and from online suppliers. (See Resources, page 126, for a list of suppliers that I trust.)

Ingredients for Herbal Treatments

Many of my recipes involve mixing essential oils into a base or carrier oil, which is then rubbed into the feet and sometimes calves. Other recipes use a powder or alcohol base to "carry" the essential oil to the feet. Essential oils are quite concentrated and powerful, and most of them should be diluted before being applied directly to the skin. All recipes in this book that include essential oils have been diluted according to safe use guidelines. For more information on using essential oils, I recommend my book *Stephanie Tourles's Essential Oils: A Beginner's Guide.*

Base Oils and Butters

As the name implies, base oils and butters serve as the base, or foundation, for many herbal products. The liquid oils called for in this book are sweet almond oil, castor oil, extra-virgin olive oil, jojoba oil, and fractionated coconut oil, all of which have delightful properties of their own. ("Fractionated" coconut oil is the liquid form; in its usual semisolid state, it won't pour into a container.) In a couple of recipes, I recommend using oil infused with comfrey or with St. John's wort; these herbs give the remedies additional soothing and healing properties.

Cocoa butter, unrefined "virgin" coconut oil, and shea butter are solid or semisolid at room temperature, and they are used to make balms and salves. You can heat them slightly in order to melt them and then mix in herbs or essential oils.

Some balms and salves also call for vegetable glycerin, which adds extra moisturizing power, and vitamin E oil (200 or 400 IU), which stabilizes the product and extends its shelf life. Small bottles of vegetable glycerin are inexpensive and widely available. For vitamin E oil, capsules are the most convenient form to use; just pierce the capsules with a pin and squeeze out the contents.

Other Ingredients

Not all recipes call for oils or butters. Powders or sprays require different bases. Listed here are some of the common cosmetic and even culinary items that you'll need for making these types of herbal foot care remedies. Most are readily available at any large grocery store or pharmacy.

- Aloe vera (*Aloe barbadensis*) gel
- Baking soda
- Colloidal oatmeal or oat flour
- Cornstarch or arrowroot powder
- Epsom salts
- Sea salt
- Sugar, granulated or brown
- Vodka, unflavored (80- or 100-proof)
- White cosmetic clay (also known as powdered white clay or kaolin)
- Witch hazel (*Hamamelis virginiana*) extract
- Zinc oxide powder

Essential Oils

The essential oils I use in these recipes were carefully chosen for their soothing, healing, anti-infective, antifungal, or other properties (sometimes all of the above!). Essential oils have become widely available, but please take care when purchasing. Not all products are created equal, and in this case, you definitely get what you pay for.

Buy your essential oils from responsible sources that harvest sustainably and create a quality product.

(See Resources, page 126, for a list of suppliers that I trust.)

Anytime you plan to use an essential oil that you haven't used before, it's a good idea to do a patch test (see facing page) to assess your potential allergic reactivity. Just because an ingredient is of natural origin doesn't mean it is safe for everyone to use. Most folks are allergic/sensitive to something at some point in their lives, whether synthetic or natural.

- Black pepper (*Piper nigrum*)
- Cedarwood (*Juniperus virginiana*)*
- Clove bud (*Syzygium aromaticum*)*
- Copaiba (*Copaifera officinalis*)
- Eucalyptus (*Eucalyptus globulus* or *E. radiata*)*
- Frankincense (*Boswellia carterii*, syn. *B. sacra*)
- Frankincense (*Boswellia serrata*)— also known as olibanum or Indian frankincense
- Geranium (*Pelargonium graveolens* or *P. × asperum*)
- Ginger (*Zingiber officinale*)
- Grapefruit (*Citrus paradisi*)
- Lavender (*Lavandula angustifolia*)

- Lemon (*Citrus limon*)
- Myrrh (*Commiphora myrrha*)*
- Peppermint (*Mentha piperita*)*
- Roman chamomile (*Anthemis nobilis*)
- Rosemary (*Rosmarinus officinalis*, chemotype verbenone or non-chemotype-specific)*
- Spearmint (*Mentha spicata*)

- Sweet marjoram (*Origanum majorana*)
- Sweet orange (*Citrus sinensis*)
- Tea tree (*Melaleuca angustifolia*)
- Thyme (*Thymus vulgaris*, chemotype linalool or non-chemotype-specific)*

***Caution:** Avoid use of these essential oils during pregnancy and while breastfeeding.

Essential Oil Safety Protocol

Essential oils must be used with care as they can be irritating to sensitive skin. To be sure that a remedy won't cause a reaction, please perform a patch test before rubbing an unfamiliar essential oil all over your feet!

PATCH TEST

Combine 1 or 2 drops of the essential oil with 1 teaspoon of base oil. Apply a dab on the underside of your wrist, inside your upper arm, behind your ear, or behind your knee, and watch that patch of skin for 12 to 24 hours. If no irritation develops, the oil is generally safe to use diluted on your skin.

FIRST AID

If you get an essential oil in your eyes or nose, immediately flush the affected area with oil (almond, olive, sunflower, jojoba, or generic vegetable oil) or with cream or whole milk. Using plain water will not help; essential oils are attracted to fats alone. Should the pain continue or severe headache or respiratory irritation develop, seek prompt medical attention. Take the essential oil bottle with you so the medical staff knows what they are dealing with.

Dried Herbs

Herbs are used in a handful of the recipes in this book. While dried herbs are far less concentrated than essential oils, if any of these are unfamiliar to you, I suggest doing a patch test to check for any skin reactivity prior to use.

- Cayenne (*Capsicum annuum*)
- Marshmallow (*Althaea officinalis*) root
- Meadowsweet (*Filipendula ulmaria*) flowers
- Peppermint (*Mentha piperita*) leaves
- Plantain (*Plantago major*) leaves
- Sage (*Salvia officinalis*) leaves
- Yarrow (*Achillea millefolium*) leaves and flowers

Herb Patch Test

Combine ½ teaspoon of the fresh or dried chopped herb with 1 teaspoon or slightly more of boiling water in a very small bowl. Let the herb absorb the water for a few minutes.

Apply a dab of the saturated herb to the inside of your upper arm or wrist area; cover with an adhesive bandage and leave in place 12 to 24 hours. If no irritation develops, the herb is generally safe to use topically.

RECOMMENDED READING

Here are some selections from my personal library of natural health and foot care books.

Bowman, Katy. *Simple Steps to Foot Pain Relief: The New Science of Healthy Feet.* BenBella Books, 2016.

———. *Whole Body Barefoot: Transitioning Well to Minimal Footwear.* Propriometrics Press, 2015.

Byers, Dwight C. *Better Health with Foot Reflexology,* revised edition. Ingham Publishing, 2001.

Dougans, Inge. *The Complete Illustrated Guide to Reflexology: Therapeutic Foot Massage for Health and Well-being.* Element Books, 1996.

Dougans, Inge, with Suzanne Ellis. *The Art of Reflexology.* Element Books, 1992.

Esmonde-White, Miranda. *Forever Painless: End Chronic Pain and Reclaim Your Life in 30 Minutes a Day.* HarperCollins Publishers, 2016.

Issel, Christine. *Reflexology: Art, Science & History.* New Frontier Publishing, 2014.

Kunz, Barbara, and Kevin Kunz. *The Complete Guide to Foot Reflexology,* third edition. RRP Press, 2005.

Norman, Laura, with Thomas Cowan. *Feet First: A Guide to Foot Reflexology.* Simon & Schuster, 1988.

Ober, Clinton, Stephen T. Sinatra, MD, and Martin Zucker. *Earthing: The Most Important Health Discovery Ever?* Basic Health Publications, 2014.

Pritt, Donald S., DPM, and Morton Walker, DPM. *The Complete Foot Book: First Aid for Your Feet.* Avery Publishing Group, 1996.

Rose, Jonathan D., DPM, and Vincent J. Martorana, DPM. *The Foot Book: A Complete Guide to Healthy Feet.* Johns Hopkins University Press, 2011.

Tisserand, Robert, and Rodney Young. *Essential Oil Safety,* second edition. Churchill Livingstone Elsevier, 2014.

Tumen, Doug, DPM. *Ask the Foot Doctor: Real-Life Answers to Enjoy Happy, Healthy, Pain-Free Feet.* Morgan James Publishing, 2019.

Villeneuve, Geraldine. *Put Your Best Feet Forward.* Balboa Press, 2017.

Vonhof, John. *Fixing Your Feet,* sixth edition. Wilderness Press, 2016.

Werd, Matthew B., DPM, and E. Leslie Knight, PhD. *FOOT!: Care, Prevention, and Treatment.* ISC Division of Wellness, 2004.

RESOURCES

Websites to Consult

American Academy of Podiatric Sports Medicine
https://aapsm.org

American College of Foot and Ankle Surgeons
https://foothealthfacts.org

American Orthopaedic Foot & Ankle Society
https://aofas.org

American Podiatric Medical Association
https://apma.org

The Foot Collective
https://thefootcollective.com

The Gait Guys
http://thegaitguys.com

Society for Barefoot Living
https://barefooters.org

Supplies and Equipment

These are my tried-and-true favorite companies and suppliers!

Correct Toes
https://correcttoes.com
A foot health tool that helps improve toe splay, balance, and stability; stretches and relaxes the feet; and can be used to restore normal and natural foot and toe function, often relieving pain and discomfort.

Eden Botanicals
https://edenbotanicals.com
Wholesale essential oils, CO_2 extracts, and absolutes for aromatherapy, natural perfumery, and body and facial care; superior quality.

Frontier Natural Products Co-op
https://frontiercoop.com
Large inventory of essential oils, packaging supplies, base oils, organic herbs, teas, spices, cosmetic clays, beeswax, and natural body care products.

Healthy Harvest, LLC
https://healthyharvests.com
Organic Tuscan estate olive oil, plus aromatherapeutic facial oil blends formulated by Stephanie Tourles, olive oil soap, and more.

Herbalist & Alchemist, Inc.
https://herbalist-alchemist.com
Wide range of superior herb products: capsules, tinctures, solid extracts, herbal oils and ointments, bitters, and more.

Jean's Greens Herbal Tea Works & Herbal Essentials
www.jeansgreens.com
A wide range of wonderful herb products, herb tinctures, teas, loose herbs and spices, essential oils, beeswax, butters, cosmetic clays, books, and more.

Mountain Rose Herbs
https://mountainroseherbs.com
Organic bulk herbs, spices, teas, essential and base oils, cosmetic clays, waxes and butters, packaging supplies, herbal tinctures and health aids, natural personal care products, and more.

OPTP (Orthopedic Physical Therapy Products)
https://optp.com
Provider of innovative physical therapy, fitness, and wellness products, including tools to help relieve achy feet.

SKS Bottle & Packaging, Inc.
https://sks-bottle.com
Glass and plastic bottles, jars, and tins of all sizes.

The Original Jojoba Company
https://jojobacompany.com
Pure expeller-pressed, organic or pesticide-free jojoba oil for skin, body, and baby care. Salves and lip balms, too. Highly recommended!

Yoga Toes
https://yogatoes.com
A foot health tool that improves toe splay, stretches and relaxes tight feet, and helps treat and prevent a long list of foot conditions and toe deformities.

Shoes

These are a few of the companies that manufacture shoes that promote healthy foot function and movement, while preserving the natural shape of your feet.

Alkahest Leather
https://alkahestleather.com

Duckfeet
https://duckfeetusa.com

Earth Runners
https://earthrunners.com

Leguano Shoes
https://leguanoshoes.com

LEMS
https://lemsshoes.com

LUNA Sandals
https://lunasandals.com

SOM Footwear
https://somfootwear.com

Vivobarefoot
https://vivobarefoot.com

Xero Shoes
https://xeroshoes.com

Some Common Conversions Used in This Book

US	METRIC (LIQUID / DRY)
1 teaspoon	5 milliliters / 4 grams
1 tablespoon	15 milliliters / 15 grams
2 tablespoon	30 milliliters / 30 grams
¼ cup	60 milliliters / 60 grams
½ cup	120 milliliters / 120 grams
1 cup	240 milliliters / 240 grams

ACKNOWLEDGMENTS

Much gratitude flows to the following folks who shared their wisdom, experiences, talents, expertise, and willing feet to help bring this book to fruition:

First, my grandfather, the late Earl C. Ashe, for introducing me to the benefits of lifelong foot care.

Deborah Balmuth, Storey's publisher, for her continued faith in my writing abilities; Deb Burns, for asking me to update my original foot book, *Natural Foot Care*, and give it new life; Lisa Hiley, editor extraordinaire.

The late William Rossi, DPM, for his refreshing and insightful views of the human foot and its care, and my amazing, uber-talented teachers Bill Flocco, Ko Tan, Myra Achorn, Geraldine Villeneuve, Vicki Graham, Karen Ball, the late Dwight Byers, Claire Guy, and Mauricio Kruchik.

Finally, all my clients, friends, and family, who've trusted me with their precious feet—to both treat and learn from—since 1988, when I worked on my first pair of feet in a spa on Cape Cod, Massachusetts. The feet do indeed reveal many, many stories!

INDEX

CARE FOR YOURSELF
with More Books from Stephanie L. Tourles

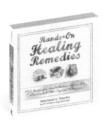

Hands-On Healing Remedies

Make your own all-natural balms, liniments, creams, and blends for a wide range of ailments, from arthritis to warts.

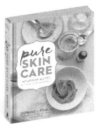

Pure Skin Care

Maintain radiantly healthy skin with 78 simple, all-natural recipes for facial cleansers and scrubs, masks, moisturizers, and steams—plus creams, balms, and exfoliants for the entire body.

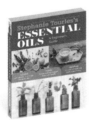

Stephanie Tourles's Essential Oils: A Beginner's Guide

Learn how to use essential oils safely and effectively! Boost your mood, relax your body, and invigorate your mind with these 100 simple recipes.